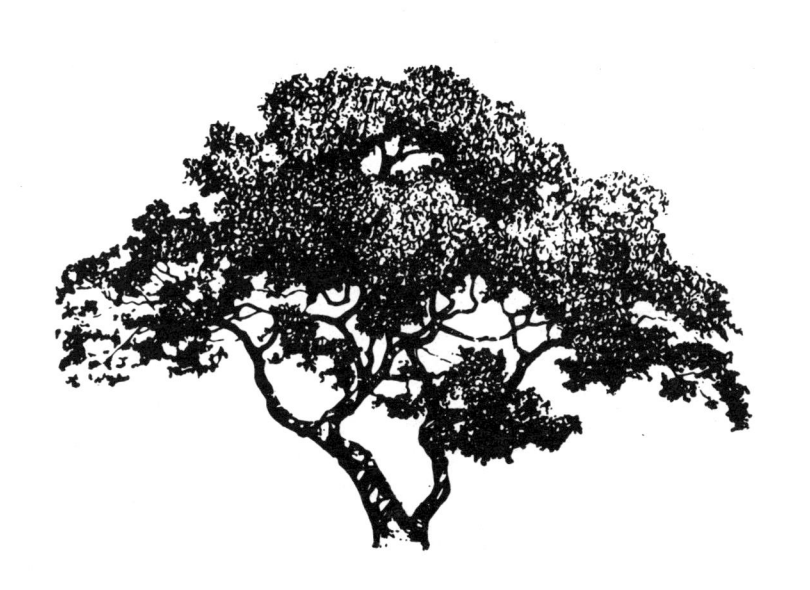

When a Friend Is Dying

A Guide to Caring for the Terminally Ill and Bereaved

EDWARD F. DOBIHAL, JR.
CHARLES WILLIAM STEWART

ABINGDON PRESS / NASHVILLE

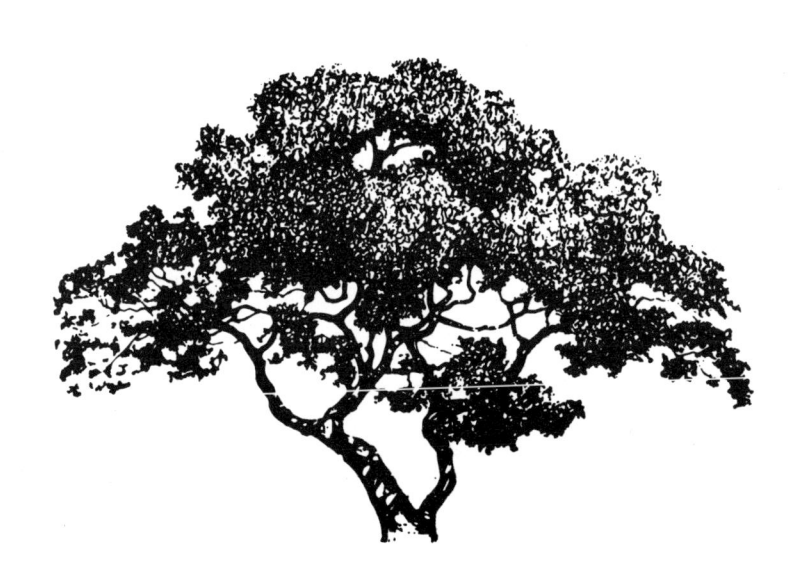

When a Friend Is Dying:
A Guide to Caring for the Terminally Ill and Bereaved

Copyright © 1984 by Abingdon Press

All rights reserved.
No part of this book may be reproduced in any manner whatsoever without written permission of the publisher except brief quotations embodied in critical articles or reviews. For information address Abingdon Press, Nashville, Tennessee.

Library of Congress Cataloging in Publication Data

DOBIHAL, EDWARD F., 1927–
  When a friend is dying.
  Bibliography: p.
  Includes index.
  1. Church work with the terminally ill.
  2. Church work with the bereaved.
  I. Stewart, Charles William. II. Title.
  BV4460.6.D62   1984   259'.4   83-15626

ISBN 0-687-44972-3

The lines on page 25 are from "Do Not Go Gentle into That Good Night" by Dylan Thomas, *Poems of Dylan Thomas*. Copyright 1952 by Dylan Thomas. Reprinted by permission of New Directions Publishing Corporation; and J. M. Dent, publishers of *Collected Poems* by Dylan Thomas.

Scripture quotations, unless otherwise noted, are from the Revised Standard Version of the Bible, copyrighted 1946, 1952, © 1971, 1973 by the Division of Christian Education of the National Council of Churches of Christ in the U.S.A. and used by permission.

MANUFACTURED BY THE PARTHENON PRESS AT
NASHVILLE, TENNESSEE, UNITED STATES OF AMERICA

*To Shirley and Alma and
Our Families*

Contents

     Introduction.. 9
    I. The Needs of the Dying............................ 13
   II. The Needs of the Grieving........................ 39
  III. The Church's Care of the Dying
       and Their Families................................. 54
  IV. The Church's Teaching About Death
       and Bereavement................................... 77
   V. A Case Study of a Grieving Family
       by Mary R. Ebinger................................ 96
  VI. The Church's Response of Preparation
       and Prophecy.. 114
 VII. Training the Laity for a Caring Ministry:
       A Training Module............................... 130
VIII. Outline of a Death and Dying
       Seminar.. 160

IX. Developing a Grief Support Group
    by Dora Elaine Tiller...............................180
Epilogue..201
A Living Will....................................205
Bibliography.................................... 209
Film Resources............................... 215
Index...219

Introduction

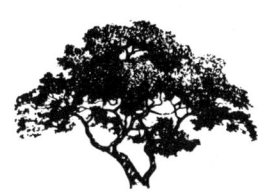

There is a quiet revolution occurring throughout the world in the care of the dying and their families. Coping with loss and bereavement are once again lively issues in our society. Dr. Elisabeth Kübler-Ross, a psychiatrist, has been an untiring worker and a prolific writer in the field. Her books, articles, and workshops have reached millions. Dr. Cicely Saunders, a pioneer leader in the hospice movement, has written and lectured to people from all over the world. She continues to demonstrate a new kind of care for the terminally ill at St. Christopher's Hospice in London. Mother Teresa has quietly led dedicated lay people and her order of nuns in ministering to the needs of the dying in India. Dr. Josefina Magno, after a bout with cancer, became an organizer of hospices in Washington, D. C., and northern Virginia and was selected as the first executive of the National Hospice Organization. Their compassionate messages of concern and care for the dying and the bereaved have slowly begun to be heard. This book is for those who want to respond. It is designed to help us look at our dying loved ones and neighbors, and at death, and teach us to be more helpful ministers at the time of bereavement.

In the western world of scientific medicine, death is still the enemy to be defeated. Life is still to be preserved at all cost. But very recently our thinking has begun to change. The growing hospice movement offers a new type of care to persons who are terminally ill and to their families. For many this has meant less personal discomfort, more personal dignity, and less money spent on care. All are vitally important factors.

We hope this book will help the church take its rightful place in assisting the dying and the bereaved. Pastors and congregations can assume important roles in assisting the growth of the hospice movement and assuring that its high principles are upheld. We can dare to include death in our life of faith; we can support one another in this final stage of our journey. This is an exciting mission of healing to which we are called.

We believe the Protestant and Roman Catholic churches are currently recognizing lay people for their broad contribution to the caring role within the congregation and the community. Lay academies and various liberation movements among women and minority groups are putting laypeople in touch with ministries to which they have rightfully been called. Holistic care centers are being established for the treatment of the total person and for the prevention of illness—for helping individuals grow toward health and wholeness. Volunteers are now participating in all fields of health—in particular, the new hospice movements. Pastors are now seeing their role evolve from primary caregiver in the parish to the professional who trains laity to carry on ministry within both the church and the wider community. In this book we provide a church and community guide for lay and professional workers who have some responsibility for the care of the terminally ill and their sorrowing families.

Each of us will write several chapters. Ed Dobihal will discuss the needs of the dying, the church's care of the dying and their families and its response of preparation and prophecy, and will outline a course on death and dying. Charles Stewart's chapters cover the needs of the grieving and the church's teaching about dying and bereavement, and also include a training module for laypeople in the care and counseling of the dying and the bereaved. Two counselors will present live case material: Mary Ebinger will discuss her pastoral care of a family in which a thirty-year-old son is dying of cancer. Elaine Tiller writes about a bereavement group which she conducted over a fifteen-week period. At the end of the book, we have included book, film, and audiovisual resources for those who desire to develop bibliographies or training tools for their work.

It would be impossible for us to name all those who have helped us write this book—our families and others who have shared their dying, their losses, their bereavement. Ed particularly thanks his friends in the hospice field in England and America; friends and groups who helped him learn at St. Christopher's Hospice; and his colleagues, friends, and teachers, lay and ordained—particularly those with whom he shares the ministry at Yale-New Haven Hospital. Charles wishes to thank those in the hospice movement in the Washington metropolitan area and his colleagues and students at Wesley Theological Seminary, who by their support have enabled him to find time to reflect and to write on these important issues. We hope this book is of particular help to laypeople, whom we believe to be the key to the pastoral ministry of the church.

> Edward F. Dobihal, Jr.
> Charles William Stewart

ONE

The Needs of the Dying

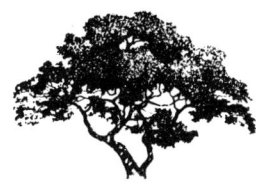

In the literature on death and dying, the phrase *the process of dying* has become common and is equated with Dr. Elisabeth Kübler-Ross' "stages" of dying.[1] Persons who experience sudden death experience no process other than living until they, in an instant, cease to live. For me that is the most fearful death, since at this moment or while driving home, it could happen to me. Also, I as a helper, in such a situation am robbed of an opportunity to help. I am robbed, that is, if I as a pastor with a congregation, have not considered dying and death as part of the normal life cycle—if I with my congregation have not thought through and felt through death and dying while alive and well.

"Chaplain, code 3, code 3, please call one, nine, six, zero." For a hospital chaplain this is a familiar sound, coming from a pager he or she carries or over the audio call system in hospital corridors. It is a common event in a hospital day or night, but each time the chaplain hears those numbers he or she knows it is an uncommon event for some person and family. The emergency room is calling so that a ministry will be immediately available to a critically ill or injured person, or to a family that is about to be told its loved one is dying, may be dying, or is dead.

All too frequently in this medical center death occurs with no time for a process of dying. This is devastating to a surviving spouse, to parents, siblings, and all others in the blood and social family. Something in them dies, as well as the person they love.

The chaplain, after a ministry of minutes or hours, determines that the family has a safe way home, since a person in shock or hysterical is not a safe driver, even if it means the chaplain provides the transportation.

Whenever possible, contact has already been made with the family's pastor. It is hoped that pastor, that congregation are prepared to provide the community in which grief can be lived out.

Sudden Death, An Important Lesson

I have stressed this type of death because so much of the writing on death and dying is focused on the terminal care of individuals who die over a period of time. We will get to that, but we will not use that phenomenon to deny another basic fact: One minute you can be alive and apparently well and the next minute you can be dead. There are heart attacks, massive cerebral hemorrhages (strokes), and automobile, motorcycle, and other accidents. As humans, we are not very fragile, but we are clearly finite, and that can be evident in an instant.

Most of these kinds of deaths occur in an acute hospital, or at least the person is pronounced dead there. That's a place we are all grateful to have in our community and a place we stay away from as much as possible. I've often heard comments such as, "You work in the hospital. That must be depressing. It's a great place when you need it but I hope I never do." Since 71 percent of deaths in the United States occur in institutions—chiefly acute hospitals—and since we tend to keep our distance, that is obviously one way we have kept distant from death and dying. Also, many of us have a fantasy-like faith that hospitals are places of modern miracles that will defeat death. Transplants, plastic hearts, kidney dialysis, nerve stimulation, chemotherapy, radiation therapy—all are, in a way, "miraculous" advances achieved within a few decades. They do often extend life and that is very good. Sometimes they extend dying and that may be very bad. They do not eliminate death and that is very factual.

Perhaps, by being willing to look at, reflect upon, and experience the anxiety of confronting sudden death, pastors and congregations can begin to prepare to minister to those who are dying. The anxiety occurs when we dare to acknowledge, "Tomorrow I may not be." Ernest Becker states, "Of all things that move man, one of the principal ones is his terror of death."[2] It may be that we cannot envision our own deaths totally, nor do we want to dwell on death in a morbid way. However, if we have not written a will, considered a living will, thought of what our absence would mean to others, then we may be too denying of our own finitude. Being too eager to help others with their dying could be a subtle part of that denial. Acknowledging my own finiteness, and my fear of that finiteness, is essential to the empathy that allows me to minister to another who is dying in his or her own way.

In summary, the sudden death does not give others an opportunity to assist the dying—only the bereaved. But facing the fact of sudden death may help me to face my finitude. That is essential if I am to help others.

Longer Dying and Death

The heading is very general as to time, since we may be speaking of days, weeks, months, or years. It becomes specific when we apply it to an individual person and family. It is important to be specific, to prevent us from placing unique human beings in a new category, "the dying," as we tend to do when we speak of "the elderly," "adolescents," those in "mid-life crises," or "doctors," "clergy," "lay people," and so on. To categorize (a useful tool at times) the dying creates the danger of stereotyping them and stereotyping an approach. This robs persons of their dignity as persons, their uniqueness and worth, and their right to live life to the end, with help, in the manner they choose. That is a primary goal of ministering to or serving individuals who are dying—to enable them to choose and to protect their rights to choose the quality of their life to its very end.

Physical Needs

Because of medical advances in surgery and the control of infectious diseases through new drugs, many of us will survive long enough to develop one or more chronic conditions. One could say that advances in acute medicine have introduced the era of chronicity. By definition, a chronic illness cannot be cured; it can only be controlled.

The hospice programs have been helpful in raising a new stage of health to our consciousness—terminal illness. An individual's health may first have been intruded on by an acute disease. For this disease all known and available medical treatments were attempted, but the disease was not cured. The advance of the disease may have seemed to cease, it may even have seemed to retreat, or gone into remission, a controlled state, but it has not gone. The individual is chronically ill and medical treatment continues to control the advance of the disease.

With life-threatening illnesses the ability to cure or to control the disease may reach its limits. Prognosis is poor, the person is expected to die, and too often the physician thinks, whether stating it or not, "There is nothing more I can do." That is true only with reference to the disease, but unfortunately we are very disease-oriented in health care. It is not true with reference to the person who is ill. Certainly the care of the person should be stressed even while focusing on the cure or control of the person's disease. But when the physician determines a person to be terminally ill, the care of that person is primary. The focus of that care must begin with physical assessment and treatment to manage the patient's distressing symptoms and provide the highest degree of comfort possible.

Physical care is primary for terminal care, but even with the advances in knowledge of symptom control gained by hospice physicians, that knowledge is not widely disseminated among physicians, nurses, and other care-givers. Moreover, this kind of knowledge is often resisted since it means developing new perceptions, a new definition of symptoms, and a new approach to both.

Since I am not a physician and since this book is not designed to be a technical statement for health care-givers, I will not attempt a detailed discussion of the physical care methods utilized for symptom control. References to excellent articles are included in the bibliography for physicians, nurses, and others who desire that technical knowledge.

However, all of us are fearful about some primarily physical aspects of dying. Will I be in pain? What if I choke to death? How weak and how much of a burden will I be, and for how long? We also hear these statements: "I don't want to be kept going by a lot of machines." "I want to die. I just want them to let me go."

The physical symptoms we seem to fear and that make us desire death include pain, respiratory distress and choking, bleeding, loss of bowel and urinary control, increasing physical weakness, and loss of physical attractiveness in a variety of ways—body odor, weight loss, loss of hair, and so forth. The effect of these losses and the other symptoms involve us in psychological, emotional, and spiritual needs, but first the symptoms must be seriously addressed by physical care.

Persons who are terminally ill and in great pain are not good candidates for counseling, casual visiting, or joining in reflection and prayer. Their prayer all too frequently is, "Oh God take the pain away." "Oh God let me die." God is not responsible for the pain or for removing it. But we are, and there are means of doing so, at least to levels where, in the majority of cases, the pain is tolerable if not all gone. Not to use these methods means, most often, that we are ignorant of knowledge in the field of pain control and/or we are resistant to change and new perspectives—and that means we are contributing to cruelty, not care. We, the recipients of health care, have the right to demand that the knowledge of physical terminal care be available for ourselves and our neighbors.

Emotional Needs

I think most of us live with our bodies in a relatively unconscious way. As long as my body is working right I tend to take it for granted. Also, since in my Christian upbringing bodies were somewhat sinful, the flesh weak, and the "form" a source of vanity, I was encouraged not to be too aware. Many bodily functions were taken care of in secret, and not too long ago even the change in body contours during pregnancy was a bit embarrassing to some.

On the other hand, our bodies are fairly important to us, and at different stages in our development we become quite aware of them. Perhaps you can remember that during adolescence you were concerned about maturing sexual characteristics or that suddenly you seemed awkward, with two left feet. Or maybe recently you looked in the mirror and saw a middle-age paunch and so off you went to a diet center. Or perhaps you suddenly saw a face looking out of the mirror that seemed strange—it was too wrinkled, the hair too gray. The new you had caught you unaware.

Those illustrations are glimpses we have of ourselves from the "outside," the awareness of change in our body through the view in the mirror. More often we think of our *internal* selves as describing, presenting, who we are. When outside changes are forced upon us by illness we suddenly find our image of ourself shattered and are aware of the damage to our internal view of ourself. To lose one's hair through medical treatment can be devastating and we want no one to see us. It would be terrible to have my body, even though I haven't thought about it much, let me down—who am I now, anyway!?

A primary need of the terminally ill—a need that is partly emotional, as well as social and spiritual—is to maintain some feeling of control over one's life. When the body is sick we are aware of it, our total self is sick, we are out of control. We need to regain some of that sense of control, and that can happen if it is clear that our wishes, our wants, our ability to participate in decisions about our life are being respected. The person who is dying, as much as possible and at least as much as wanted by that person, needs to be an active participant in the process of terminal care.

The terminally ill person also needs the freedom to engage in the process of dying to the depth he or she wishes and in his or her own time. The stages Elisabeth Kübler-Ross stated so well from her experience are emotional feeling needs: denial, depression, anger, bargaining, and acceptance. Basic to all these feelings, or emotional responses, is the fear of dying and the fear of death. Since we have been protected from a great deal of experience with dying, we are afraid or anxious about the unknowns. Also, though we have all experienced loss in life, none of us has lived through the loss of all life, which is death. Death means the loss of our entire known world and even if our faith gives us a conviction of a new world to come, the loss of the known for a still unknown is fearful.

A few years ago the question often asked by health-care givers was, "What should I tell a patient?" This assumed that patients, including dying patients, received information by what was verbally shared. That is a fairly patronizing attitude which doesn't give a person much credit for learning from the experience they are living through.

A few years ago it appeared that I would need exploratory surgery for a condition causing some alarming symptoms and which could not be definitely diagnosed by a wide array of tests. It was clear that something was wrong, but that's as far as the clarity went.

My wife and I selected a surgeon with three criteria in mind: The individual (1) must have excellent surgical skill, (2) must be conservative about deciding to perform surgery, and (3) must communicate openly with us. In our first session he agreed to answer any question either of us asked, and he added his own criterion: He would not talk to either of us separately, only together.

Among my first questions was, "Do you think I might have cancer?" My experience had led me to that fear and I was willing to state it. His response was that I might have, and he could understand the concern, but I also might have a number of other things and so he could not be definite. He also said that if he performed the surgery he would spend time with us a few days after surgery, a week after surgery, and a few weeks after surgery, so that we could ask any questions. If I asked the same question about cancer at that time, he would be able to give a knowledgeable response and he would be truthful. "I will give you time to ask but I will wait for you to ask."

Fortunately, I did not need surgery and I became well. I have often wondered whether I would have asked. Anxiety is a powerful phenomenon and I may have had to cope by not asking that question, by only commending the physician for his surgical skill and watching the ballgame with him. I trusted his perception that I had the right to denial if I needed to use that defense for a period of time.

Eventually, I would have asked, as most patients do, in either a straightforward or roundabout way. I'm sure I would then have been externally calm and controlled, internally shocked and numb, and soon quite depressed. The latter I might have been only partially aware of and would have needed others to note my changed eating habits, sleeplessness or too much sleep, inappropriate overactivity or none, and irritability as signs of my emotional state.

Those are my guesses—only that—at my response. Another person might hear exactly the same news but have a more active denial mechanism, be selectively inattentive and not hear the message at all. That person might begin to talk about how glad he or she is that the surgery is over and now all that is needed is to get well and stay that way—jogging, improved diet, church attendance, regular prayer. "This illness has really taught me a lesson. I'm going to be a better person and I know God will make me well"—a bargain.

The above illustration demonstrates that an individual, when ill with what might be a serious disease, can have a foretaste of the psychological responses present in the person who is dying. These are natural and normal responses that we have learned to utilize to cope with all of life, its good times and its crises. The fact that death is unique in that we will only live through it once does not mean we will become unique for the situation, living in a new way. One of my colleagues who ministers to many dying persons has become more and more convinced that we die as we live, and I concur.

Most of our living has been done with some degree of dependence, some independence, and some interdependence. This will be elaborated later under "social needs" but it also has implications for our psychological needs. When the balance of these factors is disrupted by hospitalization, anxiety is increased. Dependency is heightened when a person enters the hospital. Some of this is unavoidable. We must wait for the results of tests, for the results of surgery or medical treatment, and we are dependent on the authorities for interpretations and recommendations.

In my previous illustration of personal illness, my psychological needs, my emotional responses, were very real. The physician was also very present and communicating, and I developed a confident trust in our relationship. That was essential to me psychologically—it enabled me to confront the anxiety of the unknown.

In another situation, when neurological and general testing was being done for symptoms which clearly pointed to a brain tumor as one possible diagnosis, numbers of specialists were involved. A very important determinative test was performed on Thursday, with the understanding that the results would be explained on Friday. None of the specialists appeared on Friday and it is not easy in any hospital or community to obtain medical information on a weekend. This increased my anxiety and anger, which stemmed from fear but focused on being isolated by the physicians, less in control, more dependent, and less confident that the helper was dependable.

It was learned, through angry persistence, that the test was somewhat suspicious but that there were also questions about its accuracy and that it was to be repeated. This was not good news but the result for me was a decrease of fear and anxiety, and an increase of hope. The emotional needs of patients, particularly the dying, are not helped by avoidance and isolation. The message given by isolation, whether true or not, is hopelessness and that the care-givers are too apprehensive to be present.

One of the greatest fears of dying persons is that they will die alone. This fear can be heightened all through the time of treatment and care by the inconsistent presence either of those important to the individual's personal life, such as friends and family, or of those important because they are giving the essential health care. Consequently the dying person may never accept the fact that he or she is dying. Dylan Thomas speaks for many:

> And you, my father, there on the sad height,
> Curse, bless, me now with your fierce tears, I pray.
> Do not go gentle into that good night.
> Rage, rage against the dying of the light.[3]

However, the dying person may accept dying and death if he or she continues to feel physically cared for, accepted, supported, and loved.

Social Needs

Most people have families with some members close at hand and others a phone call or letter away. If they don't have families, many have colleagues and friends at work, or in the retirement center or church community. But even though some have no families or friends, most people have human contact through going to the grocery store for food, the drugstore for medicine or tobacco, or the newsstand for a magazine or daily paper. We may feel very independent but it is clear that we relate to others in many ways, we are part of humankind, we are social beings. We decide how much we will be involved with others, and that varies from a hermitlike existence to a life that is crowded with other people. That is our choice. What does it mean when we are dying?

As already stated, one of the greatest fears of dying persons is that they will die alone. Increasingly there is another fear being expressed; that they will die in the strange surroundings of a hospital or nursing home. Both these fears are statements about another segment of life which we are accustomed to controlling—our social *milieu,* people and places.

Since we usually are in control of life, or think we are, at least, we sometimes are not aware how often we are told by subtle and not so subtle means the way life should be lived. Television is a great advocate of the good life, the social life with friends and families that is the backdrop for commercials, from air travel to beverages to cars. Those As, Bs, and Cs mean sociability. Also, if we eat the right health foods and vitamins, jog in the right footwear, take the right drugs, and use the right cosmetics, we'll stay young, lively, and look and smell good enough to be the life of any party. We don't even have to worry about future security, if we'll only listen carefully to the right stock broker, have the right money-market account, bank I.R.A., and even our trip to the hereafter will be eased if we've paid our social debt with the right insurance policy. By being the right kind of consumer we can control it all, and if we don't, something must be wrong with us.

It's really not surprising when I visit the sick, including those who are dying, that I discover they feel guilty for being sick, for being a burden and causing trouble for those they love and for society in general. Sometimes this is indirectly expressed with, "Why me? I've tried to live a good life and I haven't hurt anybody." We also express that guilt, along with some fear, when we deny symptoms, or hide our sickness and try to attend to work and life as usual because we're supposed to. These are the social needs that are imposed on us by the mores and values of this particular society. They add a great burden to the person who is dying and cannot possibly meet those demands.

I have stressed these factors because they increase the complexity and difficulty of social needs for persons who are dying, their families and friends, and those who care for them. This is the inclusive social grouping necessary for the dying person, and it needs to be maintained in a natural state as far as possible. It goes contrary to our current norms to be in the hospital when we are sick, for that is not a normal place. The first need is to be in the most natural place for normal social living, and for most people, that is their home.

This simple social need is recognized within the hospice movement and therefore home care is primary. A criterion for hospice programs stresses that care be provided at home for as long as appropriate. The very seriously ill, terminally ill person, may want to and may be able to stay at home until death. Medical and nursing care can be provided in the home with family and friends assisting. Those loved ones also provide the support and the inclusion in family living that gives meaning to the person who is anticipating leavetaking but has not left. But the family and friends will need to be included by the professional care-givers; they need to be taught what they can do, be supported and encouraged, and be affirmed in the fact that they are doing what is appropriate. The latter factor is very important. This is an anxious time, and families may wonder whether they should turn to the mecca of health care, the hospital, or even better, the medical center, where "they can do so much more." At this stage in the process of dying those places cannot do nearly as much as the properly supported family. That is difficult for both professional care-givers and family caring persons to acknowledge.

However, it may be impossible or inappropriate for the person who is dying to remain at home. It would be inappropriate if the sick person did not want to stay there. It would be impossible if there were no family or friends to provide sufficient support, and professionals were unable to be present as much as necessary. It would be inappropriate if the family were simply unable, for physical or emotional reasons, to meet this very demanding situation. In this latter case, if the family could accept its limitation or did not want to provide such care, then resorting to the hospital or nursing home might not be too difficult. However, if it were an elderly wife who had come to the end of her physical resources, or even had become sick herself because of her efforts to serve her partner, then she might feel very guilty and berate herself for her failure.

If dying persons must be in a place other than their own home, they still have the need to control their space and their interactions with other people as much as possible. Since in an intensive care unit this is impossible, it is hoped the professional staff is enlightened enough to know that such an environment is inappropriate for a person who has been declared terminally ill. In other sections the hospital team may verbally say to a patient, "This is your room." But by their behavior, members of the team usually imply, "We were only fooling, this is still our place you know." For example, I don't know many hospital rooms that include a Do Not Disturb sign. Quite the contrary, too often the staff views a closed door as a swinging door. Entry is without a knock, a function may be performed without an explanation, and the intruder may not introduce himself or herself, even though a stranger.

Dying persons do want and need social interaction but they may withdraw through apathy or sleep when their decreased energy does not allow them to cope with the busy assertiveness of others. The dying person (others as well) needs to be able to say, "Not now" or "Could we talk a bit?" or "Could I eat a little later?" or "Can you come back for my tray in a little while? I couldn't eat that fast" or "Would you sit with me while I eat? I hate to eat alone." The social interaction may be wanted at a particular time, not wanted at another time, and the pace may need to be slower. Caring for the dying person means flexibility, not a rigid routine, if social needs are to be met.

If the dying person has neither family nor friends, the interactions with staff are even more primary. These are the last persons on earth whom he or she will share life with. It may be important to reminisce, to learn something of the nurse's life beyond nursing, to develop social ties that then are relinquished. Caring for the dying can be difficult because it can become personal, and then grief is heightened for the staff.

The main social needs, however, do not involve

staff. The dying person needs to continue to be involved with his or her own life, for it is that life, the things and the people, that the person is saying goodbye to. The person needs to be asked more than once in the process of dying, "What is it you want?" Many times the answer is given in social terms, "I want to plant my tomatoes," "I want to go out to the garden." That could only be accomplished at home, but there is a basic need for many to get back outside, to see the earth and its fruits and the sky again. We may have forgotten to look at such sights today, but we "know" there will be tomorrow. Today is the important social time for the dying person, and tomorrow, when it becomes today.

It was a dying person who wrote:

> Each morning is new now. I wake to the inner music of thanks for the dear gift of life and with eager plans for the uses of the day. The first sound I hear, whether a flock of chirping birds, or the whispering wind, or of traffic with its urgency, is dear. The growing light is an omen, and a good one. Thoughts crowd in, and the mind's wheels begin their busy turning like those of the cars and trucks out on the main road.
>
> Morning has always been a good time for me; I have always awakened in eagerness to get on with the day's work. But now that I know my mornings are, like all men's, limited, even if they come to a few thousand more, they are too precious to take for granted. I must taste them, and everything, both for the first time and the last. And so should we all do, always.[4]

I have used the words *taking leave* and *goodbye* several times in this section, since that is the social task for the dying person. But not all are willing or able to perform this task. Many perform it a bit subconsciously and indirectly. Others engage the task very directly. Still others may deny their leaving totally and just die. This is a very difficult social process, for the dying person is involved in all the stress of anticipatory grief. He or she is leaving everything, including loved ones. The family and friends are being left, but left with everything except the partner, parent, sibling, friend.

The stress of dying and anticipatory grief can mobilize our good intentions to protect the people we care about from pain. Many people think they can do this by lying or by shading the truth. It is sad when a patient says, "I know I'm dying, Chaplain, but I can't talk about it with my family. They're pretending so hard to cheer me up." If a family has never been able to communicate in a crisis situation, this style of behavior is not unusual, but the normal pattern. However, if it has been a family that has shared life, then it is sad not to share in the final living of life to its end.

I say "share in the final living of life" because that is what dying is. Some people can get caught up in almost a morbid fascination with dying. A patient can become so preoccupied with dying that he or she forgets there is still more living time with family and friends. The same preoccupation can occur in loved ones who seem to treat the person as dead before death occurs. Pastors and church friends who know these people and the ways they have related can be helpful when they sense that they are out of phase with one another, interpreting the time inaccurately.

For most people there is no right time to die. Most

still have more things to do, more relationships to continue or discover, more places to see, more time to reflect and be. Some single elderly people, however, may want to die so they can renew their life with family and friends in the hereafter. Their faith is in that new future which links them with a happy past, since the present is unfulfilling. Even these folks are living out a social need as they talk about the past and its meaning and express their hope for a new fellowship in God's eternal world.

It is important to help some dying persons express their social needs and then help them attempt to meet them. The businessman may want to bring his work to an end and finalize financial matters. Often there are family events like weddings, anniversaries, birthdays, baptisms, bar mitzvahs, confirmations to be experienced. In addition there are Christmas, Passover, Easter, Thanksgiving, and all the other significant holy days and holidays. Some dates may even need to be changed. These types of immediate goals give hope and meaning to life. They make the immediate time important, and being included among the living can, surprisingly, make the leaving easier for the dying person and for the bereaved who will look back. Grief is easier when we can remember what we did and do not need to say too often, "If only I had . . ."

Spiritual Needs

The spiritual life has been involved in all that has been discussed. The spiritual life makes us whole in all of life. It connects us to our God on whom we are always dependent, to others who also are children of God, and to all creation, which is the gift of God.

Anything that wounds us physically or emotionally, or separates us socially from others and from creation, tests us spiritually. Let us look for the spiritual dimension in a few of the situations discussed under other headings.

Physical care was stressed as the beginning focus for care of the dying. The physical need for pain control was emphasized. The way this need is met can either support our spiritual well-being or further wound it. Tremendous pain can lead to increased feelings of punishment and the question thrown out is, "O God, what have I done to deserve this?" If members of the medical and nursing staff do not have an adequate understanding of the difference between acute and chronic pain and are not using the recommended methods, the pain will not be controlled. It is worse if they subtly convey a rejecting attitude or even make a direct statement such as: "You have to get hold of yourself. You've had sufficient medication and can't have any more now. What's the matter with you?" This raises guilt. It adds to the feeling of being judged and found wanting. It is punishing and further adds to the wounding of the spirit. We do not care just for the physical side, the body of the person. All who care for the dying are spiritual care-givers as well.

Under the section on emotional needs I stressed the need for the dying person to be included as a primary participant in his or her own care. When the person who is dying hears "What is it you want?" and receives care in such a way that he or she can believe those words are important, it is spiritually uplifting. It conveys the message that the person is still important, still of great worth.

Serious sickness does much to rob us of that feeling of worth. Our weakness and other symptoms may deprive us of our ability to work and do many of the things that gave satisfaction and meaning to life. Changes in physical appearance may have made us feel unacceptable. Our spirit may be crying out, wondering if we will be accepted by others, by God. To be included in the process of care, to be asked what we want, is a message of worth to the spirit.

Excellent, even expert scientific and technical care that is distant is inadequate and harmful. It contributes to the already growing feelings of being unworthy, no longer even able to contribute to our own living. The dying person needs warmth, relationships, concerned interest in order to experience "the goodness of the Lord in the land of the living."

These illustrations point to the spiritual need of the dying person to continue to feel whole. That is partially accomplished through physical-symptom management so that all energy is not consumed by a concern with the body. And it is partially accomplished by the involvement in care that helps the person emotionally to feel included and in some control. Under social needs I also stressed that many individuals want to be surrounded by the loved people important to their living as well as the loved objects of life found in their homes. Leavetaking is a spiritual need in the spiritual journey of life and they are taking their leave from specific people and things.[5]

Mr. Waddie Williams was an elderly patient in a hospice program. He was totally bedridden at home where he was cared for by his wife and his middle-aged son. The nurse who was caring for this family was concerned because Mrs. Williams, who was suffering with arthritis, was continually going up and down stairs with meals and medicine in order to care for her husband and spend as much time with him as possible. The nurse suggested a hospital bed for the patient's comfort, located downstairs for the wife's comfort. Mrs. Williams said yes to the bed, but politely and very affirmatively pointed out that she wanted Waddie upstairs, near her, where they had been together for sixty-three years.[6]

Waddie was not a very verbal person but he could convey in a few words, by his facial and body expressions, his satisfaction with how he was living his life and taking his leave. He had always been a singer and an active member of his church choir. While Mrs. Williams and the nurse made his bed and gave him physical care they often would sing gospel hymns. Waddie would join in. Both Mrs. Williams and Waddie were apprehensive when it was recommended that he go to the hospital for two nights and three days for care that could lead to his greater comfort. The fear was that he would be taken from his family's care, the family home, be kept much longer in the hospital and that he would die there.

Waddie did go to the hospital and the treatment was helpful, but he withdrew, became apathetic, and said never a word. He came home on schedule, but continued withdrawn and silent. His pastor and church choir had made regular visits to the home during the illness to sing with Waddie. They came again on Sunday, about three days after the still silent Waddie had returned from the hospital. The nurse was invited and joined the group for prayer and singing. As the hymns rang out in his room, Waddie's lips began to move and gradually he began to quietly sing with his choir. Waddie was returning to participate in life with his friends and family.

When the singing drew to a close the nurse asked Waddie if he had enjoyed it. In a strong, loud voice, he responded, "Sure did!" his first words since leaving for the hospital. It was the social setting, the inclusion by friends and family, the spiritual gift of singing the loved hymns with those he loved that brought him back to life. He and Mrs. Williams had a little more time to care for each other and say their goodbyes.

Late one evening Waddie Williams, Jr., telephoned the nurse to tell her something was wrong with his father. Could she come? The son met her at the door and she went upstairs to the patient. Because death seemed imminent, the nurse called Mrs. Williams. Mrs. Williams came and cradled her husband in her arms. The nurse asked if she might pray and Mrs. Williams said, "Oh please!" The nurse gave thanks for the life of love the Williams had shared, for the gift of Waddie's life, and she asked God to receive him and care for him now. During this prayer Waddie's pastor arrived and joined in this conversation with God with strong amens. The wife sang the loved hymns, "to sing Waddie across" as he quietly died. A year later, on an anniversary bereavement call, Mrs. Williams was still grieving, but she declared that the prayer had sustained her through it all. "I know he is all right. I know he heard you. God must have sent you. I know he did."[7]

Not everyone, including those who are terminally ill, is an active participant in the religious community as Mr. Williams was. Nor does everyone who has not been active in religious life suddenly become interested in it when he or she becomes terminally ill. Dying people's needs for dignity and wholeness, for reconciliation within themselves and with important people in their lives, their needs for acceptance and forgiveness, for feeling they belong and are loved may be expressed as secular rather than as spiritual needs. It is hoped that the care-giving will seek to meet these needs in a faithful way, even though faith in God does not appear to be an explicit part of that care.

Many persons, however, at some time in their history, have had a relationship with the church. They may have drifted from participation. Perhaps there was an incident or series of incidents that caused them to become alienated from the religious community. They may feel that separation with great anger, great sorrow, or both. These folks may want to talk about their fractured religious life, their beliefs and doubts, their anger and sorrow, their desire to relate to God in a meaningful way. They may talk first with a nurse and, indeed, may want to share their spiritual needs and search only with that care-giver rather than with a minister. Other persons will ask for a minister, priest, or rabbi, to seek the possibility of a reconciliation with God within the religious community before leaving this life. For some, that seeking may be caused by their fear concerning the next life and their acceptability. In my experience, for most it is a seeking of a sense of belonging and acceptance, of peace in this life before it ends.

Those like Mr. Williams who have been active in the life of the church community need to continue to be included. They may carry on their individual practices of prayer and Scripture reading, but to be deprived of their sense of being part of the corporate Body of Christ is a great loss. Their spirits need to join others in praising God, in confession, in the joy of their faith, in song, in sacrament. This is a true testimony that they are not walking alone, that others are with them in the valley, that the Good Shepherd is truly present. In this there is hope. This is perhaps the greatest spiritual need of the dying. All care should address this need and be truthfully hopeful.

Notes

1. Elisabeth Kübler-Ross, *On Death and Dying* (New York: Macmillan Co., 1969).
2. Ernest Becker, *The Denial of Death* (New York: Free Press, 1973), p. 11.
3. Dylan Thomas, "Do Not Go Gentle into That Good Night," in *Death in Literature*, ed. Robert F. Weir (New York: Columbia University Press, 1980).
4. Bradford Smith, *Dear Gift of Life*, Pamphlet 142 (Lebanon, Penna.: Pendle Hill Publishers, 1965), p. 9.
5. Note in the Gospels the number of chapters and the emphasis devoted to Jesus' leavetaking. In the Christian calendar Lent stresses this theme every year.
6. This is a social need that is often ignored in care of the dying. Many persons want to continue to sleep together, to share warmth and affection, to engage in sexual activity when possible, and these needs are seldom provided for in the institutional setting.
7. Mrs. Williams, Waddie Williams, Jr., and the nurse, Shirley Dobihal, reviewed this brief case presentation for accuracy. Real names are used at the request of the family as an offering of thanks for the care, and as a memorial to Waddie Williams, Sr.

TWO

The Needs of the Grieving

Families begin to grieve when the doctor tells them a loved one is terminal. We have been discussing the needs of the dying patient as he or she confronts death. Now we will examine the needs of the grieving individual and/or family after the loved one has departed. What is the nature of the grief process? How can a care-giver understand bereavement so as to render the best help? How does it vary from the death experience for the individual and the family? How can we understand what loss does to the griever and to the family so that both may be given support throughout the experience? Finally, what happens in an actual family? We need to learn about such an experience so that we can understand grief from the inside.

Grief—Its Nature

Basic work on grief was begun by Sigmund Freud in his paper *Mourning and Melancholia*.[1] Freud distinguishes between a normal grief experience and an abnormal one. In the former the individual mourns the loss of a significant person and, because the mourner has a healthy ego, is able to work through the grief process fairly quickly. The melancholic, on the other hand, has a fragile self, is unable to work through the loss, and thus experiences depression or other psychotic or neurotic illness. Freud studied grieving among psychiatric patients and saw it in relation to his libido theory. For him it involves *decathexis,* unloosing the investment of psychic energy in the lost one, and *recathexis,* investing that energy in someone else. The anxiety and insecurity recapitulates the loss of the mother in childhood (age 4 to 6). Melanie Klein placed the period of loss earlier—in the first year of life, when separation anxiety over loss of the mother is deeply set in the unconscious mind.[2]

In England, John Bowlby's epic work on *Separation and Loss* challenged Freud's conclusions as to how the grieving process originates.[3] Bowlby believes the loss experience relates to the child's formation of a perceptual world. Separation anxiety occurs, however, as the child masters the anxious world, particularly as he or she gains autonomy and develops a self picture with its various components (the empirical self, the active self, and the looking-glass self). Loss of any kind triggers the individual to set up behavioral patterns to restore proximity to the loved object. When this fails, the child perceives its constructed world to be in danger and becomes insecure. The child's crying, pining, and restless activity are for the purpose of restoring the lost object. When the loss is permanent this behavior becomes redundant and senseless but that does not prevent it occurring.

Colin Murray Parkes, who has worked with John Bowlby and also with the Harvard Project, is able to bring a lot of research together in his writing. "Grief," he says, "is a process of realization, a making real the fact of loss" inside the self, an event which already has occurred in reality outside.[4] In his research on widows and widowers on both sides of the Atlantic, he particularly emphasizes the social side of grief. The griever experiences a change in her or his world which makes it immediately different. First there is *deprivation*. Without a mate one's needs for companionship, sex, economic security, and the structuring of time are not met. Second there is *social stigma*. The community looks upon the widow as different, not a member of a complete household and therefore not eligible for many family-oriented activities. The grief process involves recognizing the loss to one's social world as well as internalizing that loss so that one perceives oneself differently.

Social-systems thinking has enabled us to see the change in family balance which follows the loss of a significant member. If parents lose an only child they change from parents to a childless couple again. If a child loses a sibling, he or she must become oriented to the parents differently, particularly if that sibling was the favorite child. These losses involve a reinvestment of emotional energy as Freud and Lindemann have indicated. But they also involve a radical change in self-perception. Further, the loss causes a shift in family balance and structure, which causes a shift in each family member's relationship to his or her social world.

Theologically, the loss of a loved one forces us to reevaluate our world. Without the significant lost person and what I have invested in him and he in me, I must search for new meaning in my life. Most persons have some scenario in their heads as to their life, and a loss disrupts that life plan. The loss is a crisis, felt personally and existentially, and we ask, "Why me?" "Why now?" These questions, although they cannot be answered philosophically, indicate a search for meaning and an understanding of Providence in the midst of crisis. For this reason, grief is a crisis which may open us to a reevaluation of our faith and life philosophy.

Now let us walk through the grief process, understanding its normal character and the fact that although it has recognizable characteristics, each person, because of a unique personality and past history, will experience it somewhat differently. Let us imagine you are married and you have just received news that your mate has been killed in an auto accident. The stages of grief are presented on a normal cycle beginning with initial shock and numbness, disorganization of your self and world, and reorganization of self and world. Each stage is briefly described and the needs the grief stricken experience

Stage of Grief	Description	Needs	Duration
1. Shock & Numbness	Disbelief Rejection of loss Zombielike, stunned insulation against shock	To be alone Physical needs (childlike) Funeral planning	1 week or more
2. Disorganization	Physical symptoms Difficulty eating & sleeping Empty feeling Sense of panic Preoccupation with image of deceased Lack of action Overactivity Overactivity Hostility, guilt, & depression	Companionship To speak of deceased To ventilate intense feeling Acknowledge reality of loss To image oneself differently	6 months to 1 year
3. Reorganization	Less intense feelings Some peace and acceptance Better appearance Physically, sleeps better and eats better	To organize one's life despite loss To enter new relationships To make new starts in jobs, hobbies, travel New family structure	Several weeks to months

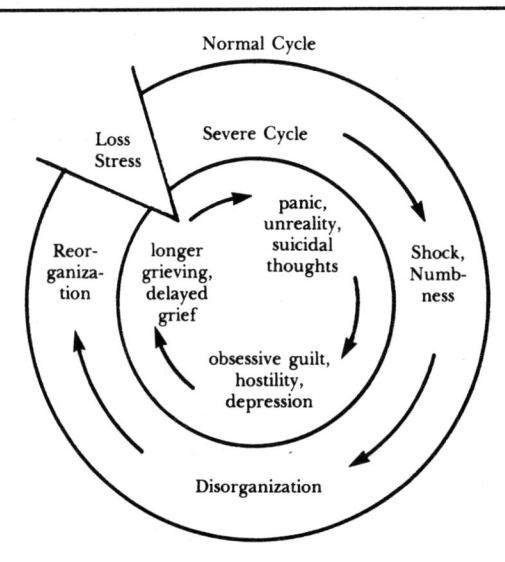

at each stage are recorded. Finally, the duration of each stage is estimated.

Shock

When news of death comes there is an emotional shock much like being hit on the head. Later that day, when one begins to realize the impact of the loss, a sense of dread and foreboding invades the consciousness. The panic reaction comes and goes in emotional waves and usually reaches a peak with the first five to fourteen days. Lindemann provides the best description from his observation of the survivors of the Cocoanut Grove fire in Boston (1943). He wrote:

> The activity throughout the day of the severely bereaved person shows remarkable changes. There is no retardation of action and speech; quite to the contrary, there is a rush of speech, especially when talking about the deceased. There is restlessness, inability to sit still, moving about in aimless fashion, continually searching for something to do. There is however, at the same time, a painful lack of capacity to initiate and maintain normal patterns of activity.[5]

Colin Murray Parkes says the principal behavior pattern evoked by loss is *searching*. When we lose a loved one it is as though we have lost a recoverable thing, like a lost wallet. We act as if we will find the lost object if we simply search in the right place. We do not believe the news. "Oh, no! It can't be," we say and protect ourself against the reality of the loss by numbness and blunting of the feelings. Grief work, says Parkes, is like worry work. "The bereaved person continues to act, in many ways, as if the lost person were still recoverable and to worry about the loss by going over it in his mind."[6]

Initially the individual, perhaps a widow, wants to be left alone, although she may not take care of herself well. She does not eat or sleep well; indigestion or nausea may be present. A zombielike appearance—even some dishevelment of clothing and slovenly appearance—reflects the loss. She needs *presence,* and to have her immediate needs taken care of. The widow needs someone to help with the funeral plans and, if there are children, to help with their care. A friend who can insist that she rest or eat will tide her over this immediate crisis period. You might not think this person is grieving, but her organism will react as though to a trauma or blow for the first week or two. It is an important stage of grieving.

Disorganization

Disorganization and despair mark the second state; the characteristic emotion the widow experiences is depression. In the early yearning phase there is *activity:* restlessness, irritability, and anger, a protest against the loss. Now that the reality of the husband's death has fully penetrated there is an attitude of defeat. She loses heart and adopts a submissive and suffering attitude. How long a woman remains depressed varies with the individual. However, recent studies of widows show that it usually lasts a year or longer. Severe grief may be experienced, as Erich Lindemann points out, as a psychotic or neurotic depression, or as alcoholism, hypochondria, phobia, or other psychosomatic illness. Certain individuals are grief-prone—that is, they have not managed earlier losses well and this loss opens an old wound. Delay in the onset of grief (beyond two weeks), prolonged grieving (beyond a year), and an inability to move beyond the disorganization stage should alert the care-giver to the need for professional help.

The needs of the normal griever shift at the disorganization stage. Without the loved one there, the widow feels her life is a shambles and devoid of meaning. She feels waves of emptiness sweeping over her and reacts with deep sighs and spells of weeping. She cannot sleep through the night and has trouble eating. She is preoccupied with the image of the deceased, and this gives way to nostalgia about her life with him. She is inactive at times, at times hyperactive, wanting to clean out closets and desk drawers. She spins her wheels a lot and is not able to think very far ahead. The future has always involved her husband and now it looks bleak without him. Normal persons report hallucinations of the lost one, behavior that on other occasions would be considered abnormal. One widow reported driving to her deceased husband's place of work, unconsciously believing she would discover him there, even though he had been dead for six weeks.

The widow at this stage needs to get back in touch with people to talk about her feelings, to sort out the impact of the loss. Unfortunately, at this sorrowing stage many of the widow's friends drop her like a hot potato. She needs to ventilate her deep feelings of anguish, her anxiety about herself and her loss. She needs to talk about the lost one and put the various incidents involving him in perspective, remembering them correctly so that they make sense, fitting them into her assumptions about the world. The strength of the feelings about the loved one needs to be *decathected,* as Freud deduced, but the widow needs to image herself differently now, as without the loved one. The memories are put away in a memory box so they will no longer haunt her; but she now must image herself as a widow, as no longer married, and as having to make it in her existence *alone.*

Freud wisely pointed out that there is ambivalence in any relationship. The one who died is both loved and hated. "Why did my husband have to die and leave me with the rearing of the children?" is a normal question to ask and it is normal to be angry at the deceased. How that anger is handled is important. If the anger is unacceptable and turns into self-reproach the individual will probably become depressed. If there was previous separation anxiety, which returns from real or imagined losses and defeats, other kinds of emotional problems will interrupt the normal grieving process. Guilt of neurotic dimension may clutter up the individual's life around the loss experience. Normal guilt will be experienced around the death of a beloved husband—she could always have made his life easier, and now that opportunity has vanished. However, if the widow continually berates herself about the things she might have done that are now out of the realm of possibility, one can suspect neurotic guilt.

How long the widow spends in the disorganization stage probably depends upon the components of the love relationship. How strong was the attachment and of what sort? How secure was the couple in the attachment? For example, was he secure and she insecure? How much did they rely upon each other; was there a certain independence in the couple, so that each did not consider the other "all"? Fusion in a relationship, with each of the couple overdependent upon the other will mean that the grief may be prolonged and difficult. So will an emotional cutoff, if the couple stayed together for the sake of the children, or if there is a lot of emotional freight that was not talked out in the relationship. Distancing from the other becomes a significant part of the working through in the disorganizing stage. Modifying one's self-image, and consequently one's social system, becomes a major part of the next phase.

Reorganization

Some time within the first six months of grieving the mourner begins to take stock of her life and adapt to the loss. "Making a new start means learning new solutions and finding new ways to predict and control happenings within the life space. It also means seeking a fresh place in the hierarchy, reassessing one's powers and possessions, and finding out how one is viewed by the rest of the world."[7] The new organization is "in spite of" the loss; in other words, the widow has had to accept the loss and the changes in self-perception and the way the world perceives her without the marital partner. The feelings of loss become less intense as she talks about them with another, writes about them in a journal, or meditates and prays about them. There is some sense of peace and acceptance of her new status as the grief work progresses to this stage. Grief stirs up feelings about her own mortality and the imminence of her own death. These may be met with resignation or worked through in terms of a faith.

Paul Tillich is the theologian who helps us understand the root of anxiety as anxiety about death. It is related, he says, to the anxiety of meaninglessness and guilt. When a loved one dies, it threatens our underlying belief in the meaning of our lives; it further makes us feel guilty, not just about what we have failed to do in relation to the loved one, but also about our alienation from God. The terror we experience as we gaze down into the abyss is the threat of nonbeing. The courage to accept our finitude is at the root of biblical faith. We must let God be God and we must accept the fact that we are human and that all our loves are finite. The *courage to be* involves the courage to accept our finitude. We rest on the laws and structures of the universe and are willing to trust our life to the Creator of all things. This is not a stoical resignation, but a life-affirming stance. We realize that in the end love is not stronger than death, but it enables us to accept our loss and to depend finally on the compassionate concern of our neighbors and the ultimate grace of the Creator.

The grieving widow begins to make new starts and to organize her life despite the death of her mate. The loved one will always be remembered but she must now set goals and begin to make plans which do not include him. The needs of the griever shift to focus on the reorganization of the individual's life. Arranging for the care of the children, finding a job for the first time, going back to school, investing her monies, perhaps selling her home and finding an apartment take much thought and decision making. The earlier grief work has enabled the deep emotions around the severance of the marital bond to be worked through. These deep feelings should not cloud the decision making and planning, but new energies should be freed for the work the widow must do both inside the home and outside it. Some widows, feeling deep loneliness without a mate, become involved too soon in a new romantic alliance. Needless to say, waiting for at least a year after the death of a husband will enable a widow to enter a new relationship with more balanced perspective.

Family-systems theory has shown that the loss of a significant figure within a family will cause an emotional shock wave from top to bottom. If the husband and father has been the dominant figure in the family, for example, his death will run through the entire family system. The wife may develop the same symptoms he had in his fatal illness; a daughter may flunk out of school; a son may act up in some way such as becoming involved with drugs. The family homeostasis has been upset, and new family structures must be worked out before the members can become reorganized after the father's death. We shall examine this in a particular family in chapter 5. To understand how an initial piece of grief work can help in this family reorganization, let us look at an example cited by Murray Bowen.

On one occasion Bowen reports that he had an opportunity to coach a father through the initial shock of losing his young wife. The couple was in their thirties and had three children, ages ten, eight, and five. A month before the father was to go overseas on a prolonged assignment, the mother died. Bowen, a neighbor, spent three hours that evening with the father, outlining for him an ideal course of action in explaining the death to the children and in anticipating the funeral in the coming days.

> I suggested that the ability of children to deal with death depends on the adults and the future would be best served if the death could be presented in terms the children could understand and they could be realistically involved in the funeral. . . . On the issue of involving the children with the dead mother, I suggested he arrange a time before the funeral to take the children to the funeral home, to remove all other people from the room, and for him and the children to have a private session with their dead mother.[8]

Later the father told Bowen what had happened. The children went up to the casket and touched their mother. They spent some time looking everything over, even climbing under the casket. The eight-year-old prayed that his mother could hold him in her arms in heaven. In the lobby the youngest soon found a smooth pebble in a planter, took it into the room, and placed it in his mother's hands, after which the other children did the same. They then told their father they were ready to go. At the funeral the older children were calm while the five-year-old clung to his father, whimpering a little. It took only a week for the children to speak of their mother in the past tense. A lot can be said for the pastoral approach of their psychiatrist friend to this family.

Conclusion

No one is quite ready for the sudden loss of a loved one, no matter how many previous losses one has experienced. Neither are we ready for the death of one with whom we have sat over a long convalescence, even though that death strikes us with a sense of relief that the suffering is over. What we have attempted to do in this chapter is to describe the nature of grief and its process. We have traced the cycle of grief through initial shock and disorganization to reorganization within the self. Grief is a normal experience and can be lived through within the period of a year. However, there are certain needs a grief-stricken person experiences which change as he or she works through each stage. The attitude of the care-giver toward the grief stricken depends upon very sensitive listening and very careful response. We are now ready to develop a strategy of care-giving both for the dying and for the grieving. This strategy can be adopted by those who wish to join in a care-giving ministry.

Notes

1. Sigmund Freud, "Mourning and Melancholia," in *Collected Papers,* ed. Ernest Jones, vol. 4 (New York: Basic Books, Harper & Row, 1959), pp. 152-70.
2. Melanie Klein, "Mourning and Its Relation to Manic Depressive States," *International Journal of Psychoanalysis* 30 (1949): 49-50.
3. John Bowlby, *Attachment and Loss,* vols. 1, 2 (New York: Basic Books, Harper & Row, 1969).

4. Colin Murray Parkes, *Bereavement: Studies of Grief in Adult Life* (New York: International University Press, 1972), p. 156.
5. Erich Lindemann, "The Symptomatology and Management of Acute Grief," *American Journal of Psychiatry* (1944): 101-41.
6. Parkes, *Bereavement*, p. 75.
7. Ibid., p. 94.
8. Murray Bowen, *Family Therapy in Clinical Practice* (New York: Jason Aronson, 1978), pp. 332-35.

THREE

The Church's Care of the Dying and Their Families

No one has reached maturity until he has learned to face the fact of his own death and shaped his way of living accordingly.

Then the true perspective emerges. The preoccupation with material things, with accumulating goods or fame or power, is exposed.

Then each morning seems new and fresh, as indeed it is. Every flower, every leaf, every greeting from a friend, every letter from a distance, every poem and every song strikes with double impact, as if we were sensing it for the first and for the last time.

Once we accept the fact that we shall disappear, we also discover the larger self which relates us to our family and friends, to our neighborhood and community, to nation and humanity, and, indeed, to the whole creation out of which we have sprung. We are a part of all this, too, and death cannot entirely withdraw us from it. To the extent that we have poured ourselves into all these related groups and persons, we live on in them.[1]

Being with persons who are dying and with their families does indeed remind us of the precious gift of life. In the rush of living, of meeting demands and expectations, carrying out today's responsibilities and planning for tomorrow, somehow the joy of living and the value of the moment may be lost. There are so many deadlines. When suddenly we are confronted with the fact that there is one very real deadline to life, the place where the line of life stops in death, there may be a new perspective that breaks into life. Time takes on new meaning when suddenly it is a lifetime that is limited. Values are reexamined. What losses will hurt the most? What will we hate not being able to take with us? What is most important to experience in this life before the time is gone?

These are the valuable gifts of questions, reflections, ideas that are raised in us by those who are dying and those anticipating their loss. The pastoral care of the pastor and the congregation needs to begin by allowing the anxieties of this subject of death, dying, and bereavement to be raised in the caring congregation—from the pulpit, in educational programs, in the youth group, women's society, young adults, and other groups. We have been isolated from the subject too long. Death has been an event ritualized in the funeral as a major event, but what goes before and what comes after that event? Death must be brought back into life if we are to receive help for living and be able to offer help to those living out life's ending.

Listening

When I walk down the street and pass someone I know, the usual greeting is a smile, perhaps "Hi," sometimes "Have a good day!" and often "How are you?" I wonder if that question originated at a time when persons would then stop and answer it seriously for each other. Now the expected response is "Fine." I find that it startles people when I say "Awful" or "Not so good." Occasionally the startling response stops the person, who says, "What's happening?" Many times the person doesn't stop and I realize she or he didn't want to hear my honesty. I always say "Fine" when I don't want the person to stop.

I wonder how we have learned to be so private with our lives, to feel we are only living up to the duty of the day when we say, "Fine!" When I as a chaplain go to see a patient in the hospital I might say, "Good morning. I'm Chaplain Dobihal. I came by to meet you. How are things today?" "Fine!" The person is in bed, has a few tubes in the arms or other places, looks ashen gray, the bed covers show a restlessness, the eyes are cloudy and anxious, and still is "Fine!" I usually sit down and say something like, "Being here doesn't seem fine to me," and then perhaps we begin to be honest and talk, with my role mainly listening.

Since we spend so much of our time being too busy for one another, not listening to one another, we need

THE CHURCH'S CARE

to consciously work at reversing the trend. Also, for pastors and pastoral visitors, it's reversing the trend of talking, even of proclaiming the gospel. From these visitors, the question most often is, "What do I say?" The beginning of calling and counseling is learning to listen, being present with a person in a manner that says we are willing to listen. We haven't come with our message already planned. We want to hear them.

Some nurses provide a great deal of ministry to persons who are dying, and to their families. The nurse who sees this as part of essential care and is in an environment where rush is the rule of the day because of too many patients, staff shortages, an acute-care time model, is usually frustrated. Dying persons need slower care. The bed needs to be changed in a more leisurely, less bustling manner, and while it's being changed, there is time for listening. A bath is a time to be enjoyed, the touching appreciated, the foot washing a sacrament, and there is time for listening. Patients may not want a bath. Their bodily cleanliness is good enough for God. The water in the basin can grow cold while there is time for listening. These are special gifts offered by nurses and other care-givers who do physical things for patients. Sometimes during the doing the patients find it less awkward to talk, are less embarrassed, so it is an important time for listening.

Because there can be a great deal of gratification in this for care-givers, it is difficult for them to give away the tasks. Perhaps that is one reason why we have cared for most of the dying in hospitals, a special place where care-givers are in control. Listening to persons who are dying and to their families has now taught us that we must modify this approach, give some of the control away, help others to give care.

Modification of the Approach to Dying Persons and Their Families

This is not a simple matter. It involves major conscious change in the process of ethical and moral decision-making about the care of persons. In simpler times, medical care was primarily entrusted to physicians and we were grateful for their power to help us. They were the only ones seen as having sufficient knowledge and insight into the mysteries of such care to make decisions. It's not so simple any longer. We now know more scientifically and can do more technologically. The results of the use of our science and technology, however, have become visible to many, such as those in the Karen Ann Quinlan case[2]—extended care facilities, including nursing homes and the increasing costs (financial, emotional, familial, spiritual) of catastrophic and chronic care. These results aren't mysteries. The media brings them into our homes regularly. They disturb many individuals, professional groups other than physicians, and physicians themselves. The movement is toward modifying practice in terminal care by reclaiming from physicians some of the responsibility for decisions about care that we as a society have given them. That leaves us with difficult questions about who bears what responsibility now.[3]

All the complexities of these issues cannot be addressed in this book. However, they are important questions to be considered by denominations and, perhaps more important, within local congregations. A section in the bibliography of this book lists source material in the field of medical ethics, statements written by faith groups and denominations, and autobiographical material. Part of preparing for pastoral care of the dying and the bereaved is to read and confront these issues in dialogue with one another. We are responsible as the people of God. We need to confront our responsibility in the area of terminal care and bear with one another that responsibility for life.

Another important modification in the approach to the care of the person who is dying is the acknowledgment that the person is dying. This is not easy for one who has been trained to diagnose and cure disease and thus protect a person's life. A physician caring for a dying person recently said to me, "My sole purpose is to save life." He could not accept the dying person's death without fighting to prevent it. Death for him meant he had failed. He could not care without attempting to cure.

As a result of these situations, denominational bodies and secular bodies have constructed "living wills."[4] Lay people have experienced so many tragically difficult deaths that they are searching for a way to say "No!" "Not for me!" "Not for my loved one!" This is a way of saying we bear a responsibility for our care and that we want that responsibility recognized. This vital modification in approach is being stated and also is being resisted, which illustrates that modification or change is not easy.

This is an area for congregational discussion, for

listening, and for individual choice. People need to begin to say what they want—not only within themselves, but aloud to others so it can be heard and recorded. They need to say it when they are well, with the knowledge that they can change their minds when they are ill, as long as they are conscious and competent to make decisions. They also need to say it to their families. If possible, the individual and the family should select an advocate other than a family member. Such an advocate would then be able to speak for the dying, if the person cannot speak, and for the family.

This could be the beginning of clergy/congregational pastoral care of the dying—and that includes all of us, no matter how well we are today. I often think of Cain's question, "Am I my brother's keeper?" (Gen. 4:9). When I look at the Gospel direction to love myself and to love my neighbor I know the answer is yes. So it is important for us in our care of one another to establish the forums where we can say to ourself and share with others what we want in our dying. That is my/our responsibility. Others can then minister to me/us in love. This is basic to modifying the care of the dying since it begins to focus on changing control by regaining and retaining some power and responsibility for ourselves.

Control

"Mrs. _____, what is it you want?" is a question often asked by hospice physicians or nurses or clergy as care is given to the terminally ill. The care-giver listens carefully for the answer and helps patients sort through a number of answers, which can then be addressed in care. This gives back some control to the sick person. It says that what she or he wants is central and that a goal of the care is to meet the person's wishes and needs, as self-defined.

It is extremely important for pastoral care-givers to ask this question, "What is it you want?" since unless the ill person is in a hospice program, nobody else may be asking it. It is seldom asked in the hospital setting. There it is assumed the patient came to be cured, to solve a particular physical problem, and tests and treatments begin on that assumption. It's hard to say and be heard, "I want to be made more comfortable and to be allowed to die in some peace." That goes against the mores which demand cure.

This is why I stress the need to discuss these matters when you are well. If you have made out a living will privately and placed it in a desk drawer, it is useless. The living will is not a legal document, but a communication document. It provides a very important way for you to communicate with your family or other loved ones, your pastor and church friends, your physician (essential), and possibly your lawyer. The will as a document is far less important than the communication it creates. Your wishes, if you become seriously ill, are then not unexpected, not a surprise, but are part of ongoing communication which allows you to change your mind, make modifications appropriate in the present situation, or maintain your position.

When the pastor or church visitor asks, "What do you want?" and hears in response, "I want to be made more comfortable and to be allowed to die in some peace," the process of learning from the patient has only begun. If we haven't trained ourselves to hear this kind of statement, if it makes us anxious, we may try to falsely assure or support the individual. We make responses like, "Oh don't worry about that, John, you're going to get better" or "You shouldn't think negative thoughts, John, they'll only upset you and your family. Let's pray together for your health." Even if John isn't going to die, he thinks he is and wants to talk about it—so listen. If he is going to die and we tell him we're too anxious to listen, who will hear him? Will God hear? Will his faith help if we can't be with him in faith?

In fact, few persons who are dying will answer our question about their wants in the way I have suggested. If they're in the hospital they may say, "I want to go home." That's the place where they would be most in control. They would be surrounded by the familiar, the people and things they love and are saying goodbye to. They can sleep in their own beds, perhaps with the partner of many years. They may want to get out in their garden or sit on the porch or patio. The loved dog or cat will be the familiar friend who keeps them company. Watching the children play, being visited by the grandchildren, sitting around the dinner table, having a snack—all become possibilities.

Most persons who are dying, whether they acknowledge that they are aware of that fact or not, want to die at home. It is difficult, if not impossible, even for a person with a very caring family, to do so unless there is a health-care team for assistance. For the person who is seriously ill and the family to achieve this level of control, both must be taught to care as well as receive care.

Helping Others to Give Care

Caring for others is not always easy. However, we do receive gratification from being care-givers, unless we are very overly dependent persons. If someone stops us on the street, asks us for directions, and we can supply the right answers, we feel good. If we are able to send a contribution to a worthy charity providing for the sick, the oppressed, the hungry, the handicapped, the poor, we feel good. If we encourage a child to learn to take the first step, to talk, to avoid the hot stove, to learn to swim, drive, or make a responsible decision, we feel good. Let us be thankful that for most people there is a drive not only for self-actualization but for helping and caring for others. We humans do need one another to live, even though the independent, pioneer existence is currently being emphasized. There is even the scriptural statement that "it is more blessed to give than to receive" (Acts 20:35*b*). But what do givers do if there are no receivers, and how are we mutually engaged in giving and receiving?

For many people—most of us, probably—it is easier to be a giver than a receiver. It's a sign that we are O.K. Often heard in the hospital is the comment that a doctor or a nurse (I'd add a chaplain) is the worst patient. That's because they can't give up the giving role, the controlling role, to receive.

When we are engaged in the process of a person's dying—the person, the family, the care-givers—we are involved in a very unique, individual journey, and a journey that involves us all. It is important for us to become a team, to be open in our communications with one another, and to be willing to share the care-giving roles. The dying person is the primary member of the team. After all, it is that person's life we are concerned about.

This may sound very simple, but think about the times you have been sick. Haven't those caring for you done many things for you with the unspoken assumption that they know what is best for you? Certainly if you've been in a hospital you know that the schedule is regulated according to the needs of the staff and institution, not necessarily according to your desires. You may want to sleep, but you must get up early for a test. You may not be hungry, but the tray with your lunch is placed in front of you. We're all willing to put up with this for a few days, with varying degrees of frustration and anger, if we can then go home where we have more command of the situation. The person in the hospital who is not going home, but Home, may need to be given more command for those last few days and weeks.

Even if a person goes home, there probably is still a schedule of some sort. The person who is dying but doesn't want to upset the family may be able to express to a pastoral visitor that this is abrasive. You may hear comments such as these:

Illustration 1: "I can't keep up with the pace around here any more. Everybody is in such a hurry." Maybe the pace has increased because of anxiety and the family and patient need you to help them talk about it. Maybe it only seems so because the patient's perception has slowed down. That, too, the family and patient need to be helped to talk about.

Illustration 2: Perhaps the patient says, "I hear everything going on out there but they keep me here in the room and do everything for me. I appreciate all they're trying to do and I don't feel too good sometimes, but I just don't want to feel like a burden." Again there is need for the pastoral visitor to help the communication between the patient and family and to discover suitable ways for the patient to become more involved in the mainstream of family life.

Illustration 3: More often a patient who has come home from the hospital weak, depressed, in some physical discomfort, will crawl into bed. The pastoral visitor may find the person uncommunicative, apathetic, and withdrawn, or he or she will say, "Well it's all over. Yep. It's all over. I can't do nothin' more." Your cheerful denial, words of encouragement, or pep-talk probably won't change that mood. Neither would your agreement: "Yep, it looks like it's all over. Let us pray." Again communication with the family and with the patient and family together is important. Depression is certainly understandable but is it true that it's all over, that there is nothing more to do, nothing more to say, no more life to be lived? That's doubtful and probably there is a need to point this out rather than to give a simple response of sympathetic support.

Illustration 4: The pastoral visitor might find a different kind of patient lying in the same bed, however, at the next visit. The mood has changed and now the person says, "What did you come back for, to gloat? You gonna tell me how good and loving God is? Maybe he is for you, but he sure as hell ain't for me. Stop bothering me and leave me alone." It's hard to stay with someone in the middle of that anger and if he or she keeps telling you to get out, then you should go. It is the patient's wishes that are important. But you also need to say that you'll be back, and you need to come back and to keep coming back, even though the person refuses to see you for awhile. The person can be just as angry at family members, at the doctor, and at the nurses. But they are doing things that need to be done and though he or she may make their life miserable for awhile, they will not leave. The pastoring person is the only one the patient can command. The fact that you respect the patient's wishes conveys respect. The fact that you return demonstrates that the patient has not destroyed you, has not been unacceptable to you and that you continue to care.

There could be many more illustrations but they would never be sufficient to cover each person and each unique situation. Pastoral care-givers do need to know, however, that their care begins with the person who is dying. That person is grieving and is expressing that grief in some way. Elisabeth Kübler-Ross has described five stages she has observed in her work with the dying: denial, anger, depression, bargaining, acceptance.[5] People do not move through these stages sequentially, nor necessarily experience each of them, nor do they finish with one never to have it reoccur. But all the stages are important, and anyone seriously considering pastoral visits to the dying should be well acquainted with her book and its case material.

Pastoral visitors particularly need to think about how their own faith and religious practice might create difficulty in each of the stages:

Denial—We usually like people to be pleasant, to be reassured and confident even in the midst of trouble, to be strong in their faith. The person who is dying may appear to be all these things, being subtle, not blatantly saying "I'm not sick" when we know differently. We may be taken in by denial.

Anger—On the other hand, we may be taken aback by anger. Anger isn't dealt with very well in the church. It's one of those bad emotions we shouldn't have, or if we have it, we feel we shouldn't express it. Of course, righteous anger over a just cause is all right. We can be righteously angry about a lot of things, even in the pulpit, but not just angry. Being just angry is unacceptable, whereas just anger is acceptable.

I stress both, since in ministering to the dying, each of them can catch us. When the person is just angry we may say, "Now, you shouldn't feel that way." If we've had some counseling courses we might not say that. In our posture, in our facial expression, or in some other nonverbal way, however, we may decisively convey the same message. The person we're visiting, however, may express anger at dying in a disguised way. It may be anger at the doctors and the nurses for their cold uncaring attitude. It may be anger at the hospital because the room is dirty, the food is cold and unpalatable, the costs are too high. It may be anger at the family members because they don't visit enough, don't do enough, and so on. These are causes which sympathetic pastoral visitors, with their views about hospitals and doctors and nurses and uncaring families, may take up with or for the patient. When the patient is justly angry in the anxiety of the situation and the pastoral visitor tries to help, it can be destructive of relationships with the rest of the caring team, including the family. We usually do get angry at real people and situations, so it's quite possible there is some truth in what is being said. However, not the whole truth, for underneath this righteous anger is often fear and anger at death itself. That feeling may be hard to confess to a pastoral person, particularly when it includes anger at God.

Bargaining—This stage may be a favorite one for pastoring persons and one where, again, we can be taken in. Here the patient is going to do good things, is going to lead a better life, is going to acknowledge all the evil and badness of the past and turn over a new leaf. For the pastoral visitor who is very concerned that the dying person be in a right relationship with God before death, this may seem to be a blessed event. What may be missed is that the patient is bargaining so that he or she will not die. If the pastoring person joins with the individual wholeheartedly in this attitude and the person does not get better but continues to get worse, then the pastoral visitor may be seen as one who doesn't keep promises, as one of too little faith, even as a betrayer.

Depression—This stage of dying seems much more

familiar and expected, since we've all experienced loss and felt blue at times. Naturally a person who is dying is going to feel sad and it is easy to be empathetic. However, depression is a mood that is catching. One can become aware of being engulfed with patient and family in a morass of sadness that is debilitating and too soon, since there is still life to live. "Snap out of it" is not a very useful response nor is an overdose of comforting words. It's possible for patients to bury themselves too soon and it's also possible for families to act that way toward their loved ones. It becomes particularly difficult when they are out of phase—when the patient is ready for more life while the family behaves as though it were all over. The pastoral visitor and other care-givers need to look for more possibilities, more events in life, more things to be accomplished, more life to be lived.

Acceptance—This final stage is not experienced by many people. It is not a goal for the pastoral visitor, the family, or the health-care team. If a patient wants to die while still denying the fact of death, then that is more appropriate for that patient than your wish that they could be more open and accepting of the end. Also, if a person does reach this stage it may be very difficult for the family and other care-givers. When the person does accept the coming and closeness of death, then the activity, the things to do, the maintaining of relationships become unimportant. The person is letting go, becoming more solitary, moving on. The people who care will feel the distance and may want to hold on. They may find it difficult to accept the person's acceptance, for now someone they love is moving away from them on his or her own journey.

The Family

In the previous section I attempted to focus on the patient but also to indicate that the person's loved ones were an inextricable part of the whole fabric of his or her life. Care for the dying very rarely involves caring for one person. It is caring for that person and at least the nuclear social unit, for the death of one will cause something to die in all the others. Caring for the family during the time of their loved one's dying can help them after the death with their task of bereavement.

I have used two terms, *family* and *nuclear social unit*, because we need to think beyond blood relationships. Everyone dies, but not everyone lives in what we think of as the normal, congenial, supportive family. In fact, the pastoral visitor and other care-givers may discover for the first time that there has been considerable stress, strained and broken relationships, hidden life-styles, in this group of individuals. The pastoral visitor who is seeking only to be supportive, compassionate, comforting, and guiding may be surprised. The confessional calling comes to the fore when we learn of alcoholism, incest, battering, drugs, hidden homosexuality, unfaithfulness, and all the other stresses that are part of the reality of life within some social units and families. Dying is now another stress and, indeed, may bring about some reconciliation, but it can also lead to further disintegration.

Whether the dying person is in the hospital, a nursing home, a hospice, or at home, the amount of care the "family" can responsibly and effectively give needs to be considered. If they can learn to do for the person, then they will also be able to listen while they are doing in that more relaxed atmosphere. Some of the advantages the nurse receives from listening can now be realized by the family "nurses." They can learn to take temperatures, blood pressures, monitor medications, give baths, position the person in bed or chair, make safe transfers, support walking, but they need to be taught. Care-givers need to be taught, to let others assist them, and to assume independent responsibility as appropriate. This is easier at home where insurance and malpractice do not make people defensive, but it is also possible in institutions if communication builds trust among all the caring persons.

Most families want to be sure everything possible is being done for the person they love and that it is being done right. That's why the family will rush their loved one to the hospital every time there is a crisis. We have been conditioned to think that it is the only place with the only skilled people who can care for us in crisis. Certainly we would not want to be accused of failing to do all we can for our loved one. Patients and families need honest information regarding what can be done and where it can be done so they can make responsible caring decisions. If no further treatment is called for that would necessitate remaining in or returning to a hospital, the family and the patient need to know that. At the same time they need to know what ongoing care will be required to assist them to have as satisfying and as qualitatively good life as possible to its end. Excellent medical and nursing care will need to continue for the patient and family. They must be assured that it will be consistent and provide all the support they require.

This is a fearful time for most families since they are insecure and unsure whether they will have the strength and ability called for in the days, weeks, or months ahead. For the terminally ill person it is clear that the time is limited. Even so, a single elderly man or woman may not have the stamina to care for the partner alone at home even if that is wished for. There may be older children but they may not live nearby, they may have work schedules they must keep or children to be cared for. The fact that a loved one is dying is draining and terrible enough, but it brings difficult decisions and radically changes the focus and locus of life.

If pastors and church visitors maintain a close, calling relationship with the sick person and the family through times of illness they will have become part of the care-giving team essential for help. When a person is in the hospital it is quite common for pastors and church friends to visit. In a terminal situation, however, the practice of regular hospital calling is not enough. Some dying is relatively quick and may involve a hospitalization of only a few days or weeks before it is over. Pastoral care is then provided by visiting in the hospital. The church family can provide additional care by cooking some meals for the family, helping with the laundry, doing some necessary shopping or other specific task that could be helpful. But most dying is not so quick and we need to plan for other kinds of pastoral care over a longer period of time.

The essential goal is to help the dying person and the family achieve the best quality of life they want and are capable of. The pastoral visitor and church friends probably know this person and the family in their normal surroundings better than any of the health-care givers. A social worker in the hospital may have spent several sessions with these folks, gathering a social history. But that knowledge will be different from the knowledge that the pastor and church friends have gained through experience with these people over a much longer time. You may have been through other deaths with them, through births and baptisms and marriages. You have worshiped together, served on committees together, shared the Lord's Supper, and perhaps other meals around other tables. If your church has had discussions about death, grief, funerals, and such topics, then the church family and the person's family may be the only ones who have heard some of the person's views. Therefore, at least for those who have been active in the parish, the pastoral visitor begins with a knowledge of the family's history that is more than a medical history or even a social history gathered at the time of illness. You may be very helpful in assisting the patient and the family with their very difficult decisions.

Another way to help the patient and family care for each other is to encourage them and support them in sharing in the corporate life of the parish. The person may be weak, needing the assistance of a cane, crutches, or wheelchair, but still be mobile enough to attend worship, to go to a committee meeting, to attend a social gathering. These can be meaningful and nurturing events of life, but we may need to help individuals overcome their hesitancy about continuing to participate with others. They may be fearful of a physical collapse, of becoming sick in public. Changes probably have occurred to their bodies due to the illness and perhaps they have lost their hair due to the treatment. This is not easy to face and they undoubtedly would feel some awkwardness, embarrassment, fear of how others would accept them and what others would say. If the person has been visited by members of the church family in addition to the pastor, then it is hoped he or she has experienced a number of caring people in the home, and it may not be so difficult to join with them outside the home.

However, for those who are terminally ill, a time usually comes when they are confined. This may be at home, in the hospital, a hospice, or a nursing home. Individual visiting, usually by the pastor or priest or rabbi, will often continue and many times includes a sacramental ministry. Too often, however, this is seen as a private service for the patient and perhaps one or two family members. Some of the minority churches have helped me to see the value of other members of the corporate Body gathering around the person and family when they are where they can no longer come to the usual place of gathering. One does not need to leave the church precipitously if the church is truly the people, the moving Body of Christ inclusive of all, and not just a place where worship occurs. Many significant acts of life are carried out within this corporate Body, and it is important to see whether any of those events need to be lived out by the dying person before death. Is there to be a marriage, a baptism, a confirmation? Is the person waiting for Christmas,

Easter? The calendar may need to be changed, usually moved up a bit. The service may have to be adapted slightly, but participation in this meaningful life event may be what the dying person is waiting for to say amen to life.

A Lesson and Gift from the Dying

It is not easy to confront the subject of death in the abstract; it is much more difficult to confront death personally as it comes to those we love and reminds us that it will someday come to us. But as Bradford Smith said, "No one has reached maturity until he has learned to face the fact of his own death and shaped his way of living accordingly."[6]

Assisting the dying and those who will be bereaved may help us to shape our own lives differently. Suffering and pain are part of life. We may learn to stand in the midst of that real life with others, with God, and discover a peace that truly does pass our understanding. Dying persons will force us to slow down in our ministry of caring and then we may wonder why we are rushing through life. We will be forced to reflect on the meaning and value of life as God's children, meaning and value that is no longer sought or found in productivity. Rather than trying to earn salvation through works we may discover the mystery of grace abounding. When we are washing someone's feet, helping them to slowly eat, remembering the important events of life with them, sharing the pain of leaving or the anticipation of arriving, we may discover that when two or three are gathered together God's presence becomes very real. God is no longer distant, but for those moments very present and part of the prayerful conversation.

The communion of saints can be strongly sensed in this ministry, though we may not be audacious enough to consider ourselves saints. However, it can be a time of mutual caring and sharing, a time of mutual ministry. As one dying person said to me a long time ago, "Don't worry, Chaplain. Now that I have known some love in my life I'm not afraid. God will continue to care for me. I'm going home." I have always been grateful for her ministry to me.

Notes

1. Bradford Smith, *Dear Gift of Life*, Pamphlet 142 (Lebanon, Penna.: Pendle Hill Publishers, 1965), p. 6.
2. Joseph Quinlan and Julia Quinlan, with Phyllis Battelle, *Karen Ann* (New York: Doubleday & Co., 1977).
3. Tom L. Beauchamp and LeRoy Walters, *Contemporary Issues in Bioethics* (Encino, Calif.: Dickinson Publishing, 1978), pp. 286-346.
4. Appendix contains an example of a living will.
5. Elisabeth Kübler-Ross, *On Death and Dying* (New York: Macmillan Co., 1969).
6. Bradford Smith, *Dear Gift of Life*, p. 6.

FOUR

The Church's Teaching About Death and Bereavement

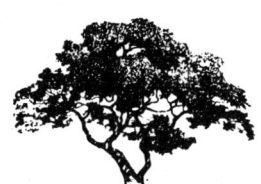

The pastor often relates in the shepherd role to the parishioner who is going through the grief experience. In a similar way the congregation, as a caring and supporting group, comforts the afflicted person and family. There are many ways the church performs a spiritual ministry to the dying and the bereaved, but perhaps the most prominent is in its preaching and teaching. There the message of the Christian faith is announced in ways which can be appropriated and accepted. Here we will examine those particular aspects of the Christian faith that meet the needs of the dying person and the bereaved in their particular crisis. And further, we will look at a particular ministry which can make the experience of approaching death and loss a more meaningful experience—namely, the life review process.

When one examines the Scriptures, one immediately notices certain significant themes relevant to the death and grief experience: the theme of loss, the theme of suffering, and the theme of the hidden God. The minister may encounter these themes if the church follows a lectionary where certain readings recur year after year. On the other hand, it may be appropriate to lift up loss, suffering, and bereavement themes at the time of a significant loss within the congregation, or when the nation or world loses a significant leader. Let us examine each of these themes in turn and relate them to spiritual ministry.

The Theme of Loss

All of us lose things from time to time. It is a universal phenomenon. When we lose something, part of the self is lost. It may only be the loss of our keys or our purse with all our charge cards. However, this may drive us to distraction. Jesus begins his stories of lost things with the parable of the lost coin (Luke 15:8-10), a small thing, but which, when it is found, leads to great rejoicing. In that same passage Jesus tells of the lost sheep and the lost son. However, from the beginning of the Scriptures, where the first couple loses paradise, on through the Bible the theme of loss is explicitly raised. People lose friends when they move, they lose jobs when they retire, they lose loved ones when they go to schools and colleges—so the theme of loss is familiar to them. The experience of loss prepares them for the experience of death.

The Experience of Suffering

The experience of suffering through sickness and injury is another recurrent theme in the Bible. Probably the suffering of the righteous is most directly dealt with in the Book of Job. Sickness, accident, and aging raise questions in people's minds about the justice of God. This is particularly so if they have some pre-Christian idea that God punishes persons by sending them sickness, injury, and bad luck. Surely people need to understand the relationship between stress and illness; however, this should be dealt with as introduction to the general question: Why is there suffering in the first place? This is a more philosophical question and should be discussed from the pulpit and in church school classes. "How could we sing the Lord's song in a foreign land?" (Ps. 137:4 NEB). This is a plaintive line from an Old Testament passage which deals directly with the suffering of the people of Israel as refugees in a strange land, bereft of their homes and possessions, but more particularly of the temple, the center of their worship and community life.

The Experience of the Hidden God

The problem at the heart of much suffering and tragedy is that the individual experiences the absence of God. It is not only that God does not seem to be just, but that he does not respond to the pleas for help. The lament psalms (for example, Ps. 22) are poems written by Israelites who felt God's absence in the midst of their trials. Job complained not only because he had lost his possessions, his family, and his health, but because God had absented himself. Elijah the prophet fled from the rage of Jezebel and hid on Mt. Horeb in a cave. He experienced God's absence and looked for a sign in the earthquake, wind, and fire. However, it was in the silence that he found God. So, too, Jesus on the cross cried out asking why God has forsaken him (Matt. 27:46). There is a "dark night of the soul," says John of the Cross, in all suffering and loss. The feeling of emptiness which the grief-stricken experience is not a proof or disproof of God. The feeling comes and goes. God's reality is affirmed on the other side of the experience of his absence.

How do the grief stricken and the dying confront the fact of loss and the riven experience of separation from those they love? The preacher or teacher should not only interpret the experience of loss, of suffering, and of the hidden God from within a Christian context, but put individuals and families in touch with the Christian faith. The two resources we want to study particularly are the dynamics of hope and of care. We shall look at each substantively as well as attempt to relate each to the sufferer in the midst of his or her own experience.

Hope

The New Testament tells us that "faith is the substance of things hoped for, the evidence of things not seen" (Heb. 11:1). There is, therefore, a close relationship between faith and hope and love, as Paul witnessed in First Corinthians 13. At this point we will deal with hope as an attitude that can be developed in the grief-stricken person.

Paul Pruyser says that hope can be defined as wishing and as the temperamental optimism which appears to be a part of some people. He makes the same distinction Ernest Schachtel makes between embeddedness affects and activity affects. Wishing, Schachtel says, is an embeddedness affect; anxiety is also an embeddedness affect. Anxiety and wishing represent diffuse tensions or discharge patterns arising from a feeling of helplessness and/or distress. The kind of thinking associated with anxiety and/or wishing is magical, not oriented to reality. The grief-stricken person, therefore, may wish that the deceased could come back to life or, out of anxiety, may move about in a distracted and distressed fashion. When one prays under such a distracted or distressed state, one may pray for a magical solution or may look to God to grant a magical answer to one's distress. Such prayer, as Rabbi Kushner has pointed out, probably will not be answered, or at least not in the way a distracted or anxious person wants.[1]

Hope, on the other hand, as an activity affect, is goal-directed and sustains optimal dimensions which enable one to satisfy one's drives. This kind of hope requires inventiveness and adapts to the distress one is experiencing. Hope, as Pruyser says, is an affect rooted in the individual's goal-directed vision and future-directed activity. One can see how this type of hope is related to faith as Paul deals with it in First Corinthians 13 and in other of his letters, such as the Letter to the Romans. The goal-directed person, one whose activity is oriented toward the future, does not cling to the past but lives in the present and is aware of the activities in which he or she must engage now. This individual is not certain of the future beyond a certain point, but courageously launches out toward that which cannot be predicted but must be trusted.

Robert J. Lifton develops five particular modes which have enabled grieving persons to face the future with a hopeful and hope-giving stance.[2]

1. Through a Biological Mode. In the biological mode one lives on through the generations of a family. One imagines at some level of consciousness that one's life continues through one's sons and daughters and their sons and daughters. Down through the generations there is an endless chain of biological attachment. This is the only kind of immortality many people can believe in. In East Asian cultures the tending of a family shrine and revering the memory of immediate parents and grandparents are ways of recognizing that one is really a product of one's parents and grandparents and that one's children will also keep one's memory alive in this fashion.

2. Through One's Creative Works. In creating a piece of art, or even through such artisan creativity as making a quilt or an end table or decorative piece, one creates something that will outlast one's own life and continue into the future. A creative writer and/or a thinker realize that such work will have an influence on human beings long past the originator's natural life. More than any other human activity, art outlives the artist. One might ask, "What does the danger of a nuclear holocaust do to this kind of hope?" Lifton raises this question in other writings—in particular, *Death in Life: Survivals of Hiroshima*[3]—and indicates that war threatens this hope.

3. Through Nature Itself. Nature preceded us and nature will outlast us, even our civilizations. In a technological society, communities tend to stray from nature's rhythms and be cut off from this kind of bond with nature. Ecologists remind us of the delicate balance between the air we breathe, the earth we live on, and the lakes which provide us with water. Scientists warn us that other creatures have become extinct when they lost their symbiotic relationship with a protecting environment. Human beings can create environments, but we will be survived by nature, and nature may cast a negative vote on some of our technology.

4. Through Experiential Transcendence. Lifton makes a great deal of the fact that individuals, through psychic states of ecstasy, can exceed the ordinary existence of the senses and of mortality itself. Within religious and secular mysticism—in the ecstasy of song, dance, battle, sexual love, childbirth—persons break the bonds of self and experience the transcendent. This may be extraordinary and lift them beyond their humdrum existence. Through athletic effort, in the experience of flight, in the perception of art and, he adds, in the drug experience, there are psychic states of ecstasy. Lifton contends this is not regression, as Freud had indicated, but a reordering of the symbolic world the individual inhabits.

5. Through the Theological Mode. The theological mode is based on life after death and is generally verified through the symbolic conquest of death on the part of the religion's hero and founder. Mohammed, Buddha, and Christ taught their disciples that the self continues in some kind of existence after death. The mystery of death and rebirth is at the center of religious conversion of the Christian. I might add that death to sin and rebirth to new life is part of the baptism ceremony. In some rituals the symbolism is acted out as persons die to sin when they are immersed and are reborn to the new life as they emerge from the water. In other words, the new life one lives by identifying with Christ gives one a foretaste of the believer's life after death.

Hope, therefore, may be seen as different from wishing. To wish for something to be different is a passive emotion and tends to lead toward wanting someone to effect a magical solution. Hope, on the other hand, is a goal-directed vision that enables one to live effectively in the present and move trustingly toward future possibilities.

Care as Love

Let's look at caring—what it means and does not mean—and link it up particularly with Christian concepts and values to see how it relates to caring for the dying and bereaved.

First, care is not sentimentality. It is not pity. When we say, "I pity you," we are keeping a person at arm's length. "I will not dirty my hands with your feelings." "I will keep you at a distance." When one pities oneself, one feels sorry for oneself. If we sympathize with another, we acknowledge the other's loss. When we sympathize, that is a little better than pity. In preaching, the preacher may overwork sentiment. He or she may use a tear-jerking example to manipulate the audience rather than to illustrate the point of the sermon. In a film titled *E.T.*, which has enjoyed a tremendous box office success, an extraterrestrial being is befriended by a boy and the sympathy of the audience is aroused. Part of the reason for the movie's success is that people feel good after a good cry.

In psychology, release of the emotions is a current fad; however, we should acknowledge the difference between *bathos* and *pathos*. Bathos involves a flood of feeling, being caught in a welter of emotions and conflict. When we care, we are not moved by superficial emotions but are open to genuine sentiment and feeling toward another.

Care is not personal domination, nor is it submission to another. When we encounter an individual who has experienced loss or is facing death, we can say, "There but for the grace of God go I." Parenthetically, we may think, "Oh, oh; I am glad this person has the crisis or the illness, not I." Care is not overpermissive. We may be so fearful of stepping on another's toes that we veer away to the other side and act like a "bump on a log." Then we do nothing at all.

When we are overpermissive we may listen to someone who has done something away out of line—that is, against our values and/or society's norms—and say nothing. When we care, however, we bring our values and norms into the context of listening, and we respond to the patient or the patient's family out of that context. Pastoral care has moved from a neutral, laissez faire position to the recognition that the caring person so greatly values the other that he or she does not want the other to live in a social limbo. As a religious counselor, therefore, we acknowledge certain values and recognize that our values will influence the way we help another.

Care is not isolation, either. Isolation seems to be a way of leaving the other person alone; letting her have the freedom to go through this process; giving her enough room. We can unconsciously move from isolation to alienation—this is certainly true in family relationships. We can give a family member freedom to grow and soon discover that we are not involved with the person at all. This noninvolvement can lead to alienation between one family member and another. The family member says we do not care because we have not come to visit for a month or six weeks or so. Caring is not leaving another alone.

Well, then, what is care? Care is not domination or sentimentality or isolation. Paul Tillich, in *The Courage to Be,* says there is a care structure in reality, that existence cares.

> Self and world are correlated, and so are individualization and participation. For this is just what participation means: being a part of something from which one is, at the same time, separated. . . . The self is a part of the world which it has as its world. The world would not be what it is without *this* individual self. . . . The identity of participation is an identity in the power of being. In this sense the power of being of the individual self is partly identical with the power of being of his world, and conversely. . . .
>
> The divine self-affirmation is the power that makes the self-affirmation of the finite being, the courage to be, possible. Only because being-itself has the character of self-affirmation in spite of nonbeing is courage possible.

Courage participates in the self-affirmation of being-itself, it participates in the power of being which prevails against nonbeing. He who receives this power in an act of mystical or personal or absolute faith is aware of the source of his courage to be.[4]

There appears to be a death and resurrection principle within nature. Scientists have discovered geological formations rising Phoenix-like out of the ashes of an earlier age that has been destroyed. Biologically, I think I am more impressed by one level of evolution growing out of another that has been, or has been proven incapable of living in a different environment. There we see the death of a species, but out of the germ cells of a previous species, like the mammoth, comes today's elephant, from both Africa and India.[5] There also appears to be *the presentiment of caring within animals themselves*. We needn't look at human beings to perceive caring between parent and child. We can see it at the zoo with the mother lion and her cub, the mother fox and her kittens. We see each nourishing her young, but we also are aware of the protective behavior of the male lion and fox.

Finally, a care structure has been established within the social structure itself. We are not talking about just pastoral care, but about human care and how it is built into the way our society is organized and the way it functions. Each of us has to care enough about what happens to the community so that we get up in the morning and go about our own little business within our own little bailiwick. If we are working in a hospital, we are under doctors' care, nurses' care, and so on, but we are also under the nutritionist's care, even the garbageman's care. All societies, no matter what their political stripe, are organized in a care structure. For things to happen efficiently, each person must assume his or her share of responsibility within the community itself. When one is unemployed or not gainfully employed, there is a sense that the society itself is not functioning in a completely holistic, efficient way.

Theologically, one finds the root of caring within the Gospel of John: "God so cared for the world that he gave us his son. . . . For God sent the Son into the world, not to condemn the world, but that the world might be saved through him" (John 3:16b-17, paraphrased). Many of us stop our thinking about Jesus with his sacrifice on the cross; we do not go on to include the rest of the passion story—Jesus' resurrection. Jesus showed his love toward both Judas, who betrayed him, and the other disciples, who forsook him at the time of his death. Jesus reveals to us a God who cares for us in our worst moments as well as our best. The gospel is about life and death and God, who takes a direct hand in our affairs. The gospel builds on the Old Testament, which is basically a story of God's covenant with his people, and the Law that directs the social behavior of the people of God. The New Testament continues the story to show us how God reveals himself supremely in the new covenant with his people. Jesus' life, teachings, cross, and resurrection all tell us about God as a caring creator and redeemer. We first understand what it means to care by acknowledging and accepting the care of God throughout every period of our lives. So when the Pharisees ask Jesus which is the greatest commandment in the Law, he replies: "Care for God with all your heart, soul and mind." This is the great and first commandment and the second is like it: "Care for your neighbor as for yourself" (Matt. 22:37, 39 paraphrased). On these two commandments rest all the Law and the Prophets.

So what does care mean? *Care means nurture and cherishing.* We not only love another, but we keep that other in a special place in our affections. To nourish is to feed and nurture another, whether as a mother with a child or as a teacher with a student. To cherish is to express a tenderness toward another, as when holding the face of a beloved. It means, "I am so interested in you that I want to promote your best interests."

Second, *Care means empathy*—that is, existing alongside another person in a dialogical relationship. The word *empathy* means to be with another, to stand with another at time of crisis or trouble. From the time of Rollo May, pastoral counselors have recognized establishment of the empathetic bond as necessary before one is able to move within a helping relationship. Buber helps us understand empathy in his book *Between Man and Man*. For Buber, empathy means "experiencing the other side." I stand with you at the bedside of a dying person. I walk with you through your grief after the beloved's death. I try to be where you are and look at the world through your eyes; hear the world through your ears; sense the world through your senses. For Buber there is no difference between the human I-thou and the divine I-Thou. Many times the only way I experience God is through my experience with my brothers and sisters.

Sometimes I hear it said that every *I and Thou* is only superficial, deep down word and response cease to exist, there is only the one primal being unconfronted by another. We should plunge into the silent unity, but for the rest leave its relativity to the life to be lived, instead of imposing on it this absolutized *I* and absolutized *Thou* with their dialogue. . . .

He experiences the cessation of his own multiplicity as the cessation of mutuality, as revealed or fulfilled absence of otherness. The being which has become one can no longer understand itself on this side of individuation nor indeed on this side of *I and Thou*. For to the border experience of the soul "one" must apparently mean the same as "the One."[6]

Compassion

The root meaning of the word *com-passion* is passion *with* or *for* another. Jesus speaks of the necessity for genuine compassion with the needy neighbor: "Greater *care* has no man than this, that a man give up his life for his friends" (John 15:13, italics added). There is a sacrificial element in caring, but it is not masochistic or self-damaging. Jesus died on the cross. We do not need to die on the cross. But by taking up one's cross one becomes a member of a servant people, all of whom care equally for one another in the way friends care for one another. This is difficult for many of the Me Generation to understand. Those with a heavy dose of self-realization psychology forget about the wounded man in the ditch, or the old person in the home for the aged, or the pensioner, or the dying in the hospice. To care compassionately for the least and the lost does mean that at times one puts aside one's own interests in order to be a member of the servant people of God. One is intentionally desirous of the best interests of the other person. One may die to self temporarily in order to rise again with the person in need.

The Me Generation is eudaemonistic in its life-stance—that is, the purpose of life is to be happy. The me-first person operates out of emptiness and loneliness. A compassionate person gives out of fullness. As the psalmist says, "My cup runneth over." One gives out of a full cup rather than an empty cup. When one's cup is lifted up and filled to overflowing by God's gracious giving, one is capable of giving to another person. Mother Teresa was asked by Senator Mark Hatfield about her goals in life. She was momentarily puzzled by his question. Then she answered, "We are not called upon to be a success; we are called upon to love."

The Life Review Process

The life review process is a way of finishing business the grieving person has left unfinished, of releasing bad memories of the past, of putting good memories into the mental storehouse. The life review process is a way of accepting what has happened at a particular place in life's journey and of consolidating the self to the point where the person is able to face the future with hope and courage. Ira Progoff, in particular, has developed a way of doing this through the process meditation and intensive journal workshops. Through these workshops on short but intensive weekend retreats, he and his colleagues have helped countless persons from various religious backgrounds begin such journals.[7] Robert Butler says that "life review marks the lives of all older persons in some manner, as their myths of invulnerability and immortality give way and death begins to be viewed as an imminent reality."[8] To review one's life at a time of crisis helps one to integrate one's self psychologically: "It is characterized by the progressive return to consciousness of past experiences and particularly the resurgence of unresolved conflicts which can be looked at again and reinterpreted."[9]

Butler and Myrna Lewis discuss several therapeutic possibilities of the life review: (1) the opportunity to reexamine the whole of one's life and to make sense of it so that identity may be reexamined and restructured; (2) the chance to resolve old problems, to make amends and restore harmony with friends and relatives; (3) the opportunity to understand and accept personal foibles, to take full responsibility for acts that caused true harm, but also to differentiate between real and neurotic guilt; (4) the opportunity to accept the reality of finitude, to mitigate fears of death and dissolution, and to develop the capacity to live creatively in the present and enjoy the moment. Says Butler:

> The success of the life review depends on the outcome of the struggle to resolve old issues of resentment, guilt, bitterness, mistrust, dependence, and nihilism. All the truly significant emotional options remain available until the moment of death—love, hate, reconciliation, self-assertion, and self-esteem.[10]

Barbara Clemons points out the relationship between life review and the confession of sins:

> The ritual and liturgy of the priestly function is not as specifically defined in the Protestant Church as in Roman Catholicism, but the function has been there nevertheless. As Butler has developed and described it, life-review therapy contains obvious elements of confession, absolution, reconciliation and affirmation.[11]

Older people experience guilt over past sins—both of omission and commission. Life review offers them the opportunity to remember the past and to get right with those they believe they have wronged. Their lives are getting short and, if they are to obtain forgiveness and make reparation, they need to do it quickly. The lay caller must be prepared for what we think of as a priestly role—hearing confession and giving a sort of absolution.

The synthesis of psychological insights into life's terminal stage of those such as Erik Erikson, Carl Jung, and Robert Butler with the insights of Christian theology has been a primary task in the current period. James Fowler contends that many adults have not grown in their religious faith but remain at an adolescent, even childish level into their later years. What he has found in his study of the *integration* to be achieved in maturity may never take place, because the individual is both morally and religiously fixated at a level of moralism (works righteousness) and conventional beliefs.[12]

Clemons sees life review as particularly appropriate for the aging person confronted with the loss in death of one friend after another. The lay care-giver should, therefore, not only expect to hear the elderly review their life story, but encourage this process. Confession will lead to absolution and reconciliation with those from whom the elderly have been alienated. Life review should also lead to acceptance and affirmation of life's journey, and a laying hold of faith in God's providence and hope in the fulfillment of God's promises. The elderly may not desire death at this point, but neither are they fearful of the termination of their life span. Serenity and a sense of peace will be the genuine attitude of such persons as death approaches.

However, some older people are able to move to a level of acceptance of their life journey with both its sorrows and its joys. Erikson speaks of integrity as involving the affirmation of this one and only life as uniquely one's own, as one looks back on the events of one's pilgrimage without regret, affirming that the journey has been good. Theologically, the Christian gains the capacity to see God's providence underlying the whole of life—despite the tragedies and inevitable setbacks suffered. The Christian is a person of hope, particularly as he or she confronts death and realizes that "nothing can separate you from the love of God"—neither life nor death.

Summary

We have been discussing ways the message of the Christian faith may be seen as a response to the experiences of loss individuals and families may undergo. Within a parish the minister, following the example of Jesus, speaks of loss, of suffering, and of grief through preaching and teaching. Moreover, a caring congregation finds ways to communicate to the grieving that hope and love may undergird them and enable them to find resources of strength and endurance. Finally, individuals may be encouraged to engage in a life review process, both at the time of death or in the experience of bereavement. The early church, according to the Book of Acts (4:32-35; 6:1-5), organized itself in order to enable the people of God to carry on a caring ministry for the dying and grieving within the congregation and community. We want now to look specifically at ways a modern group may equip itself to carry on such a caring ministry.

Notes

1. Harold S. Kushner, *When Bad Things Happen to Good People* (New York: Schocken Books, 1981).
2. Robert J. Lifton, "Five Psychologies of Hope," *Psychology Today* (November 1970).
3. Robert J. Lifton, *Death in Life: Survivals of Hiroshima* (New York: Random House, 1967).
4. Paul Tillich, *The Courage to Be* (New Haven: Yale University Press, 1952), pp. 88, 181.
5. Loren Eiseley, *All the Strange Hours* (New York: Charles Scribner's Sons, 1975).
6. Martin Buber, *Between Man and Man* (Boston: Beacon Press, 1955), pp. 24-25.
7. Ira Progoff, *The Intensive Journal Workshop* (New York: Dialogue House Library, 1975) and *The Practice of Process Meditation* (New York: Dialogue House Library, 1980) (paperback).
8. Robert Butler and Myrna Lewis, "Life Review Therapy: Putting Memories to Work in Individual and Group Psychotherapy," *Geriatrics* 29 (November 1974): 165.
9. Ibid., p. 43.
10. Ibid., p. 169.
11. Barbara Clemons, "Life Review Therapy for Older Persons: Theological Considerations," M.T.S. thesis, Wesley Theological Seminary, 1978, p. 3.
12. James Fowler, *Stages of Faith: The Psychology of Human Development and the Quest for Meaning* (New York: Harper & Row, 1981).

FIVE

A Case Study of a Grieving Family

by Mary R. Ebinger

The whole family is affected by death.

Society today may concentrate on the dying patient or on the immediate mate but not as frequently on the rest of the family. It is necessary to have not only an awareness of the dying process of the patient but the response of the other family members to this situation. The family is often neglected before death, and even more afterward.

Through the years I have become more sensitive to the needs of the family. About ten years ago I nursed my terminally ill sister in a large hospital. Not only were the patients in the cancer ward somewhat isolated by the staff, afraid of death, but the families who sat in waiting rooms or walked alone through the halls received very little care by supportive persons.

Professionally, I see many persons who must work through their grief years after a death. At the time of death the focus was on the dying patient, and the members of the families suffered in different ways.

Colin Murray Parkes of London Hospital Medical College writes about the emotional involvement of the family during the period preceding death:

> Cancer invades a family in much the same way that it invades a human body. At first its presence may go unnoticed or be suspected only by one or two members who keep their suspicions to themselves.... Just as bodily reserves are called upon in the patient himself, so his family rallies round and willingly calls upon its reserves of strength, time, money, and sympathy to support its damaged member. But just as the patient's bodily and psychological reserves may eventually become exhausted, so may those of his family.[1]

Cancer Invades Tim Johnson's Family
(All names and situations have been changed. See chart on page 99.)

Tim Johnson, a thin, stoop-shouldered boy with poor self-esteem, left home to attend college and there he became involved with drugs. After graduation he held a brief position in a department store as he "tried to find himself." Eventually Tim became motivated to become a social worker and entered graduate school. He then gave up drugs and became deeply religious. During the process of self-examination in those years he wrote the following poem.

> We are born,
> We mature,
> We see,
> We feel,
> We think,
> We love,
> We laugh,
> We eat,
> We see,
> We talk,
> We walk,
> We run,
> We hate,
> We search,
> We look,
> We plead,
> We make love,
> We make war.
> We do all the things we are supposed to do,
> And then we die.

When the Johnsons met for family sessions, it became evident that Tim had become the "good son" and surrogate father to Sally, a nurse who lived at home, but primarily to his younger brother Eddie, a teenager with epilepsy controlled by medication, who had difficulty keeping jobs and had "tried drugs" originally because of his older brother.

Tim tried to help his father understand it was not helpful to continually provide Eddie with money for cigarettes, magazines, and records. It was Tim who was the stabilizing factor between mother, father, and grandfather Joe as they talked together, blaming Eddie for his drug habits and laziness. But as the

FAMILY CHART

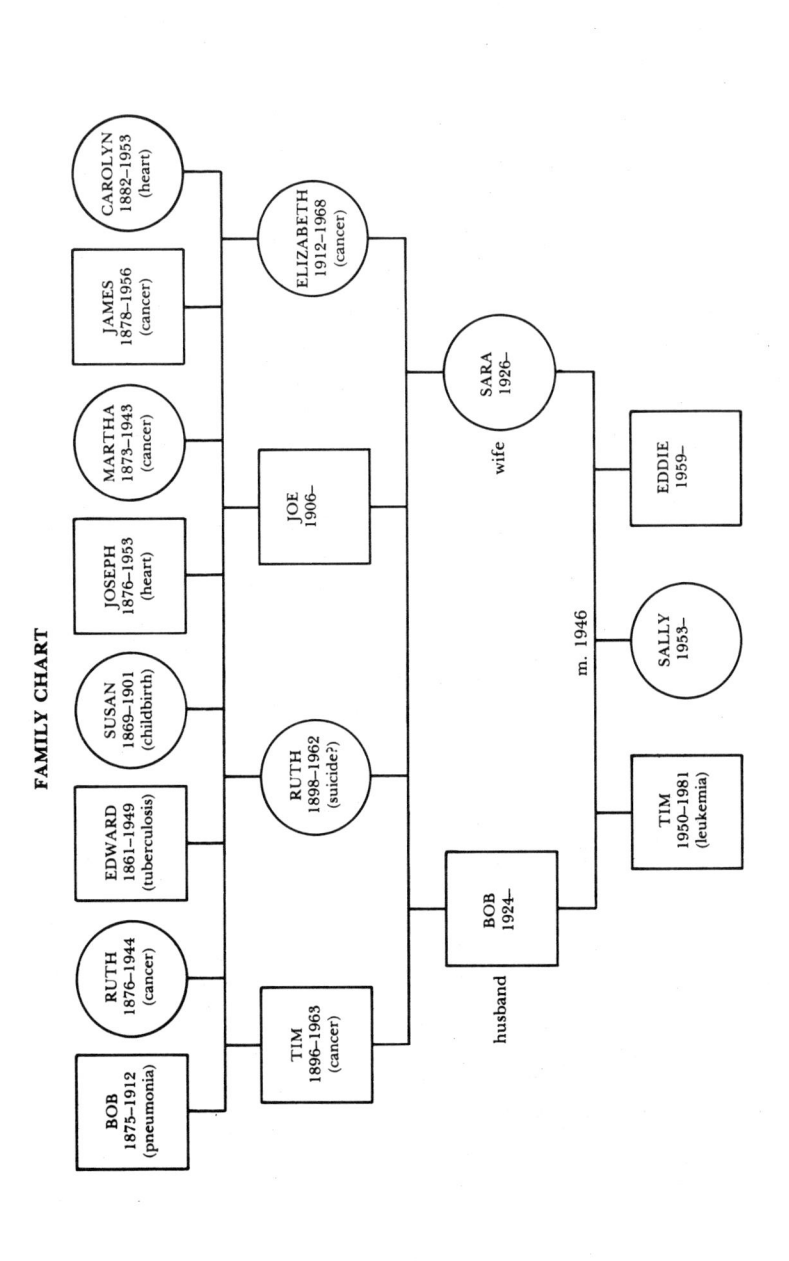

family began to work together, the focus shifted from Eddie and everyone began to communicate in a more healthy way. Eddie eventually volunteered to go into a drug rehabilitation center, and after graduation from high school he kept a responsible job in a hardware store.

At this point Tim developed leukemia. The father refused to believe the son was ill; the grandfather picked on everybody; Sally at first ignored the illness; Eddie became irresponsible in his job, lost it, and went back on drugs. Cancer was invading not only Tim's body but the emotional life of the family.

The Family's Acceptance of Death

Acceptance that a loved one is dying becomes necessary, not only for the patient, but also for the family.

In the beginning of Tim's bout with chronic leukemia, there were times of remission when he would say, "I think I am going to make it. I'm going to lick this thing. I have so much to live for." The family, too, was hopeful; it was impossible to think of anything but regained health for a person who had gone back to school and had found purpose in living.

When Tim became ill the family tried to recenter on Eddie. If Sara, the mother, tried to talk about Tim's cancer, Bob would say, "I'm sure he'll be all right. Let's not be pessimistic. What about Eddie?" Sally, too, preferred to talk about Eddie, while Eddie entirely blocked out the fact of Tim's illness. It was less painful to talk about Eddie than about Tim's cancer.

While Tim fought the cancer he also became committed to his studies in social work and his teenage cases as well as the youth in his local church.

In the meantime, Kathy, a friend of Sara, and others began to pray for Tim. There was hope that this would heal Tim. As his cancer progressed, however, Sara's friends suggested that Tim and his mother did not have enough faith. The result of this was unbearable guilt for both Tim and his mother. At one point Tim agonized to his mother, "I feel I'm a failure because God didn't heal me." The next day he said, "Mom, I didn't mean that."

His mother replied, "You are healed in mind and spirit."

Bob, the father, continued to deny Tim's illness, and more friction developed between him and Sara, the mother. Bob then moved out, physically deserting the family he had emotionally abandoned through the years. As Sally nursed other dying patients, she became depressed as she thought about her brother's cancer. Eddie slowly began to understand how sick Tim was but still tried to avoid talking about it. Each person in the Johnson family was affected. The cancer had invaded Tim's body, and also his family. Finally, they all fully realized that he was going to die.

At the point when chemotherapy, surgery, and other methods are no longer effective, it is essential that the family, as well as the patient, accept the dying process. Frequently, the patient is helped to understand this, but the family who has a dying member also needs the support and help of friends and other community resources to deal with this crisis.

Helping the Patient and Family Through the Dying Process

After acceptance, the emphasis must shift from saving life to helping the patient and family through the phases of death. Listening to the patient and family talk about the physical and mental pain and anguish is important.

Sara talked about Tim's treatment. "Tim's chest is hurting. . . . He had chemotherapy and is always nauseated. . . . He is in so much pain. . . . I know he is dying. . . . How can he bear it?—How can I?" As she repeatedly expressed her feelings with caring and loving persons, in counseling sessions, and in the cancer support group—Make Each Day Count—a quietness and peace came to her. She said, "God has helped me through the past and I feel he is giving me strength and confidence now and for the future."

As Tim thought about his approaching death he expressed himself by talking and writing about his feelings. After a hospital stay he said, "I feel like a Frankenstein monster when I have all those tubes sticking out of me. . . . I know I'm dying and there's so much I still would like to do. . . . I hope my family will be able to manage. . . . Perhaps God will use my death in some way." He wrote in his diary:

> Men have clung to their hope down through the ages. Man has always put his faith in God, himself or science. . . . The theist claims God is working in history and that his kingdom will eventually come on earth. When this hope fails, they flee to the hope that all will be put right "after death." Maybe so. Only dying will answer that question.

A GRIEVING FAMILY

One of Tim's fears was pain. He communicated this to a minister:

Tim: I am not afraid to die, but I am afraid of the pain . . . the pain of it.
Clergy: The pain of dying.
Tim: In other words, what scares me more than actually being dead is the pain.
Clergy: We haven't been able to perceive your pain. . . . You haven't been one to share pain even when people inquire about it.
Tim: I really haven't had a lot of pain, but I worry about the moments before . . . the couple of weeks before . . .

It was at this point that Tim's minister secured a doctor's help in assuring Tim that his death would be peaceful and without pain. This was true in Tim's case and he needed to express this fear and to have this assurance. Not always can such assurance be given, but the patient's fears can be learned and, to the degree possible, pain can be alleviated.

More and more, Tim began to accept his coming death. Once he put it this way: "It's a beautiful world even if you're on the way out. Whatever works out will be for the ultimate good. When I die, my spirit will be free to soar."

Sally said, "It's one thing to see people die in your nursing unit, but it's so difficult with your brother—so hard."

Eddie rationalized, "My brother can't die. . . . He won't. . . . I'm the one who should."

Listening to a family express its feelings of denial,

anger, and hurt at the death of a loved one can be helpful. The need to listen to everyone in the family is important. This can be the start of anticipatory grief for the entire family and prepare its members for bereavement. Anticipatory grief helps a family cope with reality following death. Lack of preparation tends to produce a shock reaction, but anticipation of loss diminishes shock and facilitates healing. Although a family's anticipatory grief can begin before death, it can rarely be completed at that time.

Anticipatory grief can help a family when the patient talks about funeral arrangements. Tim shared his feelings with his mother and sister. At that time Eddie still could not accept his brother's death and his father was sending humorous cards—one showed Yogi Bear laughing and saying, "It's not over until it's over." After a few similar ones, Tim did not open his father's cards. On several occasions he talked about the final arrangements:

Tim: You know I put it in my will that I want to be cremated.

Sara: You're sure that's what you want? *(tearful)* We want to do what you want.

Sally: Don't you want a regular funeral service? You don't *(choking back feelings)* want a viewing?

Tim: I don't want people seeing me like this. I really want you to get rid of the ashes in the cheapest way possible. Then I want a memorial service.

Sara: Where do you want the service? Here where you grew up?

Tim: *(tearful)* I think I'd like it at Community Church near the campus so my friends can attend, but whatever you think . . . whatever is easiest for you.

Sometimes families will say to patients, "Don't worry about anything. Let's not talk about that now. Leave everything to us." This tends to make dying persons feel helpless, whereas if they talk about the funeral plans, they feel more in control of their life even in death, and the families can work through some grief ahead of time. It is difficult but helpful to both patients and families.

Lily Pincus expresses it this way in *Death and the Family:*

> There is no growth without pain and conflict. There is no loss which cannot lead to gain. Although this interconnection is what life is all about, it is hard for those who have to face the loss of a significant person to accept. The survivor has several difficult tasks to perform. Having helped the dying to accept his death, he himself has to acknowledge the final loss of an important person and the pain this causes him and through acceptance of this pain gain strength for a new life.[2]

The Johnson family, especially the mother, found talking with Tim about the funeral arrangements painful but helpful.

Thus sharing the pain of anticipatory grief is one way family members can prepare for a new life after the death of a loved one.

Creative Living in the Dying Process

Creative living in the midst of dying can help both patient and other family members.

As Sara helped Tim entertain teenagers when he was well enough, the process of creative living continued even during the dying stages. Grandfather Joe could not understand how Sara and Tim could enjoy young people, sitting around drinking hot chocolate and eating popcorn. He commented, "I don't know how you can laugh at such a time, with all your problems and what Tim is going through!" Sara and Tim were living creatively even during the dying process.

Significant events can either unite or divide a family during this period. Sometimes a family member, such as a mother, will live until her daughter is married, or a husband who has heart problems will live until his wife dies from an illness. So Tim was living for graduation, when he would receive his master's degree in the social sciences.

The afternoon Tim was wheeled down the aisle of the university auditorium, his thin body was gaunt, his face was puffy with edema, and he was short of breath since he had become dependent on oxygen. His whole family, including his father, sat proudly though sadly in the front of the auditorium. When the time came for his diploma to be presented, Tim, with great effort, pulled himself up from the wheelchair and walked for the last time across the stage, to the applause of his family and many others who knew of his struggle. He had achieved an important goal and, moreover, it was a unifying and healing time for his family.

A GRIEVING FAMILY

The family's laughter was mingled with frequent tears as they posed for pictures with Tim. They even held a small party for his graduation. Everyone knew this was Tim's last major event. His friends and the community knew that Tim, indeed, was going to die and that he was dying in a creative way.

I talked with Tim during his last week. He was confined to bed in his home, and his grandfather and mother were replacing the oxygen tank. When they left the room, Tim requested that I move his pillow so he could rest his face on his folded hands. It was obvious he wanted to talk.

Patient:	Thank you for coming. *(silence)*
Counselor:	You seem to be having difficulty breathing. *(recognition of the patient's state)*
Patient:	Yes, it's getting harder to breathe, and it's just a struggle at this point to die. In some ways I'm ready, but there are still other things I want to do.
Counselor:	In a way you want to die but there are some things you would like to do yet.
Patient:	I'm tired of struggling, but I'd like to present a case conference yet on Jimmy who is doing so much better in school. I really feel I've helped him and wish I could share this with the staff.
Counselor:	You felt good about how you handled his case.

Patient: Yeah, but I'm still worried about Eddie. I was really the father in the family and I'm not sure I did such a good job with him. I know I didn't. It was hard being the son and father in all of this. I made many mistakes, especially when I was on drugs.

Counselor: It was a lot for you to go to school and try to be a father to Eddie, too, through all the years. You really felt bad about getting him started on drugs.

Patient: I felt horrible. I did change and tried to help Eddie then. *(talked about his father and about helping his brother enter the rehabilitation center)* I guess I did the best I could, after the drugs. Will you still see my mother? I'm worried about her.

He talked extensively about his mother and when I assured him that she planned to see me, he breathed a sigh and relaxed: "I'm glad you came." At that point, he seemed to release his responsibilities as surrogate father.

"Well done, good and faithful servant," I whispered in his ear, then kissed him on the forehead. As I prayed a brief prayer, he smiled and drifted into a quiet sleep. I never saw him alive again.

Tim chose to die in his home. His family nursed him during the last days of his life. One day when his mother had gone to the store, he quietly slipped away as if he had planned to die at that time. He handled his death in a creative way. Colin Murray Parkes writes:

> Dying is a creative act; only those who are truly alive can make something of dying. The role, then, of the dying patient is not to be a "good" patient, but to make something positive of what would otherwise be a negative event.... The "right way" for one man is not necessarily the "right way" for any other.... But we can help the patient to find his own way of dying.[5]

Family and patient can make dying a creative act, but support is needed from friends, the community, and professionals.

What Happens to the Family Afterward?

What happens to the husband or wife after the mate dies? This has been explored frequently in numerous books on bereavement. What happens, however, to other family members? The mother when a child dies? The brothers and sisters? The patient dies. The family survives. What happens to them?

Members of the family may still try to "escape" the death in various ways. Business and work may be one form of escape. Other ways may be alcoholism, drugs, suicide, and different types of illness such as ulcers, colitis, and cancer.

Let us look again at the Johnson family. Sally worked through much of her grief both with Tim personally and in the family sessions, and also in the intensive care unit of the hospital as she talked with other patients and families who faced critical illness and death. She still cried at times, but recognized this as natural. She did not try to escape her grief or bereavement.

Bob, the father, had already moved to Pittsburgh to escape Tim's death and the family's grief, denying his role as husband and father, one he had abdicated years before.

Tim's brother, Eddie, attempted suicide as an escape from grief and because he thought *he* "deserved to die" rather than his brother. What was the use, he felt. Tim had "gone off drugs," graduated, and obtained a good job. Eddie had tried to follow his brother, but then his brother had died. Another unfortunate factor was that I had moved from the area, so he also felt deserted by me, his counselor. Although he was transferred to another counselor, he could not make the transition. Recently, when I went to see him at a home where he had a rented room, he told me, "Life is tough, but maybe I'll make it." He also agreed to come with his mother for future counseling, even though the distance is greater.

How did Sara face her grief? Although she had worked through her anticipatory grief very well, she too tried to escape, to some degree, by quickly taking a job as a filing clerk in a nearby business, hired by one of her friends. She also began volunteer work with the American Cancer Society, which she said was painful but helpful as she faced those who had cancer and related to their families.

The family's balance is affected; the balance of a family frequently shifts at the death of a member. Before Tim became ill there were many different triangles, as Murray Bowen describes it in family system therapy. At times, the power was, in a sense, divided, with the father and the son Eddie aligned against the mother while the father kept the son dependent on him for money. Sally and Tim, as the "good" brother and sister, also were in a triangle, with Eddie as the prodigal.

When the family met together and interacted with one another, taking the focus off Eddie, there was a more healthy balance. Tim and Sally became independent in their own apartments and later Eddie began to function at a job.

After Tim's death Sara, grandfather Joe, and Eddie became a triangle, with Sara caring for Eddie as she had for Tim, but not to the extent of making him irresponsible, as he had been when overly dependent on the father.

What will eventually happen to this family? Perhaps Sally will become the family ideal, or maybe even Eddie. Time will tell whether Eddie will live up to his full potential. He must still be careful that he is not caught in a struggle between other members of his family, since the father still attempts to wield power from a distance. This is a simplified explanation of the balance in the Johnson family. The members continue to grieve, but much has been done to help their ability to function.

Thus we see that, following death, other family members may use various ways of dealing with the loss. Also, the balance in a family is affected. Finally, friends, members of the community, and professional persons must concentrate on helping an entire family as well as the dying patient.

Guidelines for Dealing with Death in the Family

1. The immediate task may consist mainly of letting each member of the family talk about the details of the

last deeds and days, expressing their feelings again and again.

2. In a climate of trust and acceptance, the bereaved may be able to express feelings of guilt about having failed, not having loved enough, or not having recognized the illness soon enough. In so doing, healing may occur.

3. The emotional hurts are not healed by escape, denial, pills, or alcohol—but by the listening, expressions of support, and personal concern of caring persons.

4. Attention needs to be given to small children. Do not just whisk them away because "they do not know what is happening anyway." Sometimes in later years these events return in ways that show the child felt rejected at that time. There are helpful books to explain how a child can be a part of this event in an appropriate way.

5. Teenagers need someone to listen to them, since their nonchalance frequently does not express their true feelings; they are really asking for support.

6. Members of the family who live at a distance need support, too, since frequently they cannot share in the dying process as easily as those nearby.

7. Special attention is often required by those who seem to be "handling the death so well," because later they may suffer from a lack of grieving.

8. Telephone calls and visits a week or several months later, or on special occasions, can come at a time when others tend to forget the persons or family. An occasion may be the birthday of a deceased or the anniversary of a couple—especially difficult times.

9. Grieving varies from one person to another. It is

important to realize that some hurt, guilt, or anger at the death of a person may be normal. Extreme feelings, or lack of any, however, may need additional professional help by clergy, counselors, or doctors.

The most important factor in dealing with the crisis of death is the ability of the family to adapt and refocus its energy toward the future. As Charles Stewart expresses it, "The family system is resilient and bends and creaks and groans much like the house caught in the rains and floods and winds. Whether it survives or falls depends on whether it is capable of change."[4] The success of the family in surviving the change brought by death is dependent also on the support and caring of the larger community of faith.

Notes

1. Colin Murray Parkes, "Emotional Involvement of the Family During the Period Preceding Death," in *Acute Grief: Counseling the Bereaved*, ed. Otto S. Margolis (New York: Columbia University Press, 1981), p. 23.
2. Lilly Pincus, *Death and the Family* (New York: Random House, 1976), p. 275.
3. Parkes, "Emotional Involvement," p. 23.
4. Charles W. Stewart, *The Minister as Family Counselor* (Nashville: Abingdon Press, 1979), p. 82.

SIX

The Church's Response of Preparation and Prophecy

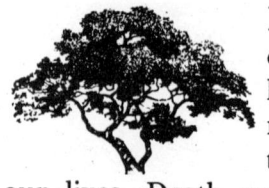

In this book we are encouraging congregations to enter into dialogue about death and bereavement, to once again allow this terribly important topic to enter our lives. Death was once a natural part of our households, experienced at home. It wasn't an event to be glorified. It brought loss and sadness and helplessness, but it was known and part of life. Too often now death is witnessed only by physicians, nurses, perhaps a hospital chaplain, and is unknown to most of us. It has become another of the medical mysteries from which we are excluded, rather than remaining a natural part of the journey of life. Willard S. Krabill has written a description of death from two health perspectives:

> *The Biomedical/Mechanistic View.* Modern medicine has reached heights of curative potential never before realized. Dying is an illness, the ultimate illness—to be treated, controlled, cured if at all possible, and for as long as possible.
>
> *The Wholistic View.* Death is a part of life—the next stage of growth. Death is a normal and natural phenomenon and is not to be resisted at all costs and by any means. There are fates worse than death. The physician should help people make decisions about the time and circumstances of their death. Death is a transformation—a return to God.[1]

We need to reflect upon the tensions created by these different views of death. It is important for individuals to choose their view, to articulate it, and to act upon the choice. It is an illusion to think that death will simply happen. More often it will follow a process of dying. Do we see that process as a disease to be treated? Or do we see that process as a normal phenomenon to be lived out as the final stage of growth, an ending and a beginning? If we have the latter view, then there is work to be done and this chapter will outline some of that work. Only when that is accomplished will change occur and will there be an option to the biomedical/mechanistic view.

The Congregation's Preparation

When the principles of hospice care being practiced in England were introduced in this country many people who were members of Christian congregations were very responsive and became early supporters and spokesmen for hospices. Many physicians were skeptical at first and some were antagonistic. On the other hand, many nurses, social workers, and clergy were interested, ready and willing to explore this new kind of care. The leaders of health care institutions, hospitals and nursing homes, were interested from a distance, but also were skeptical, waiting to see, and when they felt this care might be a threat, antagonistic.

Congregations need to understand that movements for change in the care of the terminally ill will involve conflict. One of the conflicts will be the surfacing of the tension between the biomedical/mechanistic view and the holistic view of death. Another conflict may be with current health care organizations. Hospitals, nursing homes, home care organizations, and health departments have developed their own ways of doing things. They may see hospice programs as intruders, critics of their functioning and threats to their finances.

Hospice, Inc., was founded in November 1971 in New Haven, Connecticut. The conflicts just mentioned were those that organization experienced. In addition, it learned that some geographic communities were not prepared to confront the anxieties of death and of dying persons. When Hospice, Inc., was seeking to purchase land on which to construct a facility it discovered that some communities were frightened of the terminally ill. One site was selected because it was next to a playground, in a setting with activity that would be stimulating to patients and families. Adults prepared a petition against the location of the hospice in that neighborhood. The young people who took the petition from door to door said, "You know those people's minds will be affected. Do you want them to molest your children on the playground?" Those children learned those thoughts from adults. Anxiety and fear can produce strange and irrational responses, but they are understandable. Dying and death have become so foreign to us that we want to keep them at a great distance—perhaps then they'll go away.

If Christians want their light to shine on this arena of life they need to know that many will want to turn it out. They need to know that some will want to cover that light and not let it shine to reveal the darkness that exists around death and dying. If Christians want to proclaim, "Death is swallowed up in victory. O death, where is thy victory? O grave, where is thy sting?" (I Cor. 15:54-55 KJ), then we must prepare. We must prepare not only to determine what those faith statements mean, but how we will act to develop programs that will allow us and others to live out that faith.

Within the framework of the local church there are many possibilities for examining our faith with reference to death, dying, and bereavement. Our worship certainly reminds us through hymns, prayers, Scripture, preaching, that we are living in eternal time, not just temporal time. We are a resurrection faith, constantly dying and being reborn in this life's progression through loss, grief, and the discovery of new life.

No one can develop from birth through childhood, middle age, and the senior years without loss and, it is hoped, growth at each transition. There are rites and practices of the church for most of those stages—baptism, church school classes from nursery to adult, confirmation, marriage, birth and baptism again, and the funeral. It isn't only the funeral that involves loss, though it is the rite that does confront the one total death that each of us will live through. But all those other transitions mean that we are moving from something to be mourned, to something to be celebrated. We should not celebrate only as we enter these events. The preparations for baptism, confirmation, marriage, and those that we now need to develop for the middle and later years, should include confronting and working through the losses so that we will be more realistically ready for the new.

People say, "How can I prepare for death?" Since this is a unique event that is not repeated, we cannot prepare by trial and error. Some interesting experiences are being recorded about near-death, but they are about near-death—not death. However, we can reflect on our losses, our changes, our transitions, to see how we coped with them. This may tell us something of our style of living with loss, which probably will be our style of dying.

In this process of congregational reflection to prepare us to faithfully look at death in our lives, we may discover how to helpfully include the emotional responses to life in our worship and Christian communication. Dietrich Bonhoeffer tells us:

> Nothing can make up for the absence of someone whom we love, and it would be wrong to try to find a substitute; we must simply hold out and see it through. That sounds very hard at first, but at the same time it is a great

consolation, for the gap, as long as it remains unfilled, preserves the bonds between us. It is nonsense to say that God fills the gap; he doesn't fill it, but on the contrary, he keeps it empty and so helps us to keep alive our former communion with each other, even at the cost of pain.[2]

Bereavement does include grieving, a physical and emotional response to loss/death. Though we have a strong faith, this does not mean we will not grieve or should not grieve.

> When Jesus saw her weeping, and the Jews who came with her also weeping, he was deeply moved in spirit and troubled; and he said, "Where have you laid him [Lazarus]?" They said to him, "Lord, come and see." Jesus wept. —John 11:33-35

Often, however, those who are grieving will stay away from Sunday worship and other congregational gatherings. These are times when they could receive consolation, be surrounded by their compassionate and caring sisters and brothers. However, unlike some pentecostal and black churches, in many Protestant churches we have developed worship that is filled with emotional words but stoic practice. Countless people have said to me, "I couldn't go to church today. I knew I would start to cry when we sang the first hymn." Others have been afraid they would break down when they went to the altar rail for the Sacrament. We sing:

> Just as I am, though tossed about
> With many a conflict, many a doubt,
> Fightings and fears within, without,
> O Lamb of God, I come, I come!

We may sing that we can come to God just as we are, but it seems we are afraid to be just as we are with one another.

We will need preparation to help us discover our feelings with one another. We will not all experience the same feelings or express them in the same way. However, if we are preparing so that we may practice a ministry of care for the dying and the bereaved, we will need to feel and to know how to be with others in their feelings. This is a vital part of our preparation and we may discover that it raises conflict within us and between us. But take courage, God will be present with us and with all our feelings in the midst of conflict. Living through that conflict will prepare us for the next step—a prophetic word in our community.

The Prophetic Word

Assisting Hospice to Progress. If we want options other than the biomedical/mechanistic view of death and the treatment methodology that develops from that view, let us first look to see if options already exist. Dr. Cicely Saunders brought the first message of English hospice care of the terminally ill to this country in 1963. Twenty years later it is estimated that approximately twelve hundred groups are at some point in the development of a hospice program. Every state has at least one group that has begun to investigate hospice concepts, plan a program of care, or offer such care. This is very rapid growth. With the federal legislation passed in 1982 to provide remuneration for terminal care by hospice programs beginning in 1983, the growth will become more rapid.

THE CHURCH'S RESPONSE

The new method of remuneration means a transition: The hospice movement will be brought into closer relationship with the Medicare System. I have been suggesting that every transition involves loss and gain. That will undoubtedly be so in this case. It is important that the prophetic eye be kept on the original vision which stimulated the hospice movement and that the prophetic word be spoken against any dimming of that vision through bureaucratic interference, lowering of standards, or attempts to use hospice primarily for financial gain. Those who began the movement, working hard against apathy and considerable opposition, want to keep the vision bright. They will appreciate knowledgeable persons to support them and join in that task.

If a hospice program of care exists in your community I would recommend that pastors and congregations become well acquainted with its services and needs. The persons who are in such a program can help congregations consider the issues of dying and bereavement within the church program. They can also provide information about the option for the type of care their program will offer the people of the church when they are in need of it.

Prophetic Pioneering. You may discover that this type of program does not exist in your community but that it does somewhere near, in your state or in a neighboring state. It may be helpful to visit with them, seek consultation from them as you consider the needs of your community and the program possibilities. We have become so lulled into thinking that someone else—a hospital, physicians, nursing homes—will look after our health needs that we have forgotten this is one of our responsibilities. It is a particular responsibility and mission of the Christian community. We are called to a ministry of healing. The church has pioneered in establishing general hospitals, in the mental health movement, and in providing enlightened nursing-home care. The church, local and national, should be providing leadership in this new venture of hospice care.

A local church in a local community will seldom be able to develop a hospice program alone, nor should it. The needs of a whole geographic area with its variety of people, the pluralism of religious groups, the existing health care providers and the patterns of their use, the number of deaths each year—all these factors need to be surveyed and considered in planning a program of care. This planning requires a team of individuals that includes some persons well acquainted with health care in the region—physicians (a few), nurses (including those in the public health sector), social workers, clergy (and a hospital chaplain if possible), a health planner or planners. Most needed, however, are lay and professional people who know the need for a new method of care for the terminally ill because of their personal experience. These people will be open to change, motivated to bring about change, and willing to endure the conflict that will arise. Let me emphasize again that lay people, consumers of health care, are vital to the process. They will keep the professionals from slipping into old patterns, the usual language and practices that health professionals feel comfortable with but which set them apart.

It is a pioneering venture to bring this mixture of persons together to think and plan. It will take leadership and persistence to keep them together, to help them break out of the tracks of their specialties, to begin to accept the ideas of others. Unfortunately, all of us seem to become encapsulated in our specialties and suspicious of others who seem to be treading on our turf. For example, some clergy like to think they are the most knowledgeable about and therefore are in charge of the spiritual dimension of life. They may wonder about doctors or nurses or homemakers who talk about reading Scripture and sharing prayers with patients and families. Also, others on the team might mistakenly expect clergy to handle all spiritual concerns. In another area, doctors and nurses might have some disagreements about the way they must share responsibility for medication usage. Both groups might wonder how much they can share with patients and families these responsibilities which they regard as theirs.

The disagreements, difficulty in listening to people with different backgrounds and skills, impatience, and intolerance that surface during thinking and planning reflect what will later occur in learning to work together in giving care. If a group discovers it cannot plan together, then it hardly will be able to practice together. Today this kind of planning can test itself against some helpful externals—the principles for hospice care that have been developed from the English example and from experience in the United States. Hospices vary greatly from community to community and not all terminal care will be provided by all hospice programs. But if care is to be given it must reflect the following definition or, though it may be terminal care, it will not be hospice care.

Definition of a Hospice Program of Care

A Hospice is a program of palliative and supportive services which provides physical, psychological, social, and spiritual care for dying persons and their families. Services are provided by a medically supervised interdisciplinary team of professionals and volunteers. Hospice services are available in both the home and an inpatient setting. Home care is provided on a part-time, intermittent, regularly scheduled, and around-the-clock on-call basis. Bereavement services are available to the family. Admission to a Hospice program of care is on the basis of patient and family need.[3]

After a group has determined that there is a real need to provide an option for persons who are dying and their families, they will need to consider the option of a hospice program. Do they want to construct a program that will seriously uphold the hospice definition? Will it be part of an already existing health care provider's program—the program of a hospital, a nursing home, a visiting nurse association, a collaborative effort of several agencies—or will it be a new community program? If it does become part of an existing organization or institution, how will its autonomy, its new insights and style, its unique contribution be protected and not diluted? In existing structures, there are established lines of authority and power. How will the hospice program be provided with sufficient power and authority to protect and preserve its program? These are important questions for the development of a program. The answers probably will demand skillful compromise to bring about constructive collaboration, but the goals and standards of hospice cannot be compromised.

All that has been said about the complexity of beginning illustrates why a local church probably cannot begin and own a hospice program. However, an invested local church which has a group of individuals who have seriously considered death, dying, and bereavement can initiate the discussion of hospice, can bring together people who can plan and protect the goals of care. The group will need to reach beyond itself to include other Christians (different styles), other religions, humanists, minorities, and interested health care professionals.

Education will need to be planned for this larger group and then expanded into the community. This step will lead to the discovery of other interested people who will become active volunteers and supporters. It will also educate the original group to the resistances that exist and will need to be addressed.

This is exciting work that, at times, is frustrating. In a real sense it takes the Word out into the world, where you will find that the Word is already at work. However, you must listen patiently to a variety of "languages" when you begin to talk about health care. Among the many words, it may be hard to hear the Word, to feel God's presence and direction in the process. Those Christians in the planning and implementing process may want to set times, open to all, when they can spend some quiet time, prayerful time, or discussion time, to be sure they are still listening to and communing with God about His/Her work in the world. Care needs to be taken that this doesn't become a separating activity. All will need support, and groups will need to discover a variety of ways to support each other—days away (a secular retreat), social gatherings, think together/share together sessions, celebrations. Those who find support in Christian Communion and community should not apologize for or neglect that source of faithful renewal.

What we're discussing is the potential for developing partnerships between institutions and people who are concerned with providing better care for terminally ill persons and their families. These latter and bereaved families who already have lost a loved one will want to join this partnership. In fact, when we were developing the program in Connecticut—seeking essential funds, appearing before community groups, testifying in governmental public hearings—these people were our best teachers and most moving advocates. They could state their needs from personal experience in very human terms. Hospice is partnership in care with them; it is not just another kind of health care that is done to or for them.

This kind of partnership demands the capacity to learn to blend roles in shared tasks. In the early days of the movement, we called it *blurring* roles, but that's a fuzzy term for a fuzzy practice. It is essential, for example, for each professional person to be highly qualified, competent, secure in his or her professional role. No person can do everything or totally direct everything. There are tasks that only a doctor, only a nurse, only a volunteer, only a clergy person, only a social worker can do. These tasks can be performed in a consistent and compassionate way, discussed openly with others across disciplinary lines; the views of others might be enlightening. Partnership, or teamwork, takes commitment and work. Without such an investment in working together, hospice care cannot be attained.

Leadership of the Church

I believe the church is called to take a leadership role in supporting or developing options of care for dying persons and their families. I have tried to indicate that such leadership should be toward bringing about a cooperative venture in a concern that is a local community, a societal matter.

It is not easy in this country or in any country to just give care. Unless the venture is totally volunteer, it involves hiring people, paying them, receiving remuneration for care provided, acquiring a license, meeting professional and governmental qualifications and standards, and other complex issues. If there is a hospice group in your locale, it undoubtedly needs your interest, support, help. If there is no such group, the church needs to seriously consider the need for such a program for its members and neighbors. Though the task may be complex, it is not impossible. Someone must begin, and that can be a leadership role for individuals commissioned by a church.

One of my dying friends in St. Christopher's Hospice in England said, "You know, it's good to be in this place where I belong, where I felt welcomed, where people care—even love me. A place where people have time to share with me. They're never too busy for a smile, a word, or to sit down and hold my hand, even cry with me. So you've come all the way from America to learn from us. Well, go back, and if you don't have a place like this, start one for people like me." My friend was assigning me a very serious religious mission in that conversation in 1970.

Since that time I have heard many dying persons and their families in this country asking for that kind of enlightened care. They must have excellent medical care which will address their symptoms so that they can participate in a qualitatively good life until they die. They need the support of others to help with their spiritual, emotional, social, and financial needs. We now have experience enough in this country to know that we are not talking about hospice as a *place* for such care, but as a *program* of care, designed in different ways in different communities.

We share the call to participate in that mission of creating new possibilities for care. The local church is called also to continue to include dying persons and their families in the corporate life of the congregation. In addition, the parish can develop new ways to support its members and neighbors, such as the concept of bereavement teams discussed in the next chapter.

The tasks are many and they are not easy. Dr. Cicely Saunders has said that though St. Christopher's is not a religiously owned institution, it was the religious foundation that created and supported it. The church has its faith to support it in facing the difficult. We can go forth and know that God is with us in a mission of love. We can dare to include the anxiety and fear of death in our experience of Life.

Notes

1. Willard S. Krabill, *Health: A Medical Concern,* bulletin, American Public Health Association 47/1 (Winter 1983): 20.
2. Dietrich Bonhoeffer, *Letters and Papers from Prison,* rev. enl. ed., Copyright © 1953, 1967, 1971 by SCM Press Ltd. (New York: Macmillan Publishing Co., Inc.), p. 176.
3. "Definition of a Hospice Program of Care," in *Standards of a Hospice Program of Care* (Arlington, Va.: National Hospice Organization, 1981).

SEVEN

Training the Laity
for a Caring Ministry:
A Training Module

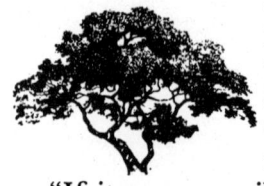

Most of us have experienced the helpless feeling that accompanies grief. "If I were just able to do something for Mrs. Brown, a recent widow," we say to ourself, or, "If it were possible for me to help this grieving parent who has lost a young child. But I don't know how." How does one move from the stage of wanting to help a mourner toward actually doing something that gives comfort and support? That is the focus of this chapter.

At the outset we have already understood that the grief stricken do not want to be alone, although they will need quiet times to themselves. Nor do those experiencing loss want to be pushed and probed beyond their capacity to handle the stage of grief they are experiencing. More than anything else the mourner wants the presence of another, even though that other is silent, merely being near through the period of deepest hurt. Howard Thurman catches that mood:

> I share with you the agony of your grief, the anguish of your heart finds echo in my own. I know I cannot enter all you feel nor bear with you the burden of your pain; I can but offer what my love does give: the strength of caring, the warmth of one who seeks to understand the silent storm-swept barrenness of so great a loss. This I do in quiet ways, that on your lonely path you may not walk alone.[1]

How does the primary care-giver train laypeople in the art of counseling the dying and bereaved? Many hospice workers have developed training modules, some relevant for urban settings, some for suburban and university settings, some for rural settings. We shall present a training module for laypeople who may be working in a church or agency setting. It is not necessary to have a college education to become a grief worker; one should simply have the gifts and graces of a caring person. However, it is our contention that even the most gifted person will benefit from a training experience. It is hoped that the lay person will become one who accepts the universality of grief, and also accepts the possibility that most persons, with help, can successfully work through that grief.

Setting Up the Bereavement Counseling Training Group

The primary care-giver, whether minister, social worker, visiting nurse, or psychologist, will want to attend to several matters involved in setting up a training group. (I am assuming that the trainer has not experienced the luxury of having someone else set up the group.) Those matters are enlistment, screening, motivation, and curriculum.

• Enlistment •

One of the primary target groups consists of those who have been through a loss themselves, have successfully managed their grief, and feel they have some insights to share. Some of these persons are capable of counseling others and some are not, as we shall discuss in the section on screening. However, many of them are highly motivated to offer help to others. Another group consists of those who are in the volunteer pool—that is, those who volunteer for many other kinds of service but who have never been a part of the caring ministry of church or the lay counseling of an agency. Others who should be available are those who are in people-oriented professions—teaching, social work, medicine, law, and so on—who could quite easily adapt their approach to people to take account of grieving. The selection team should be open to people from many areas, but it should be made plain that there will be a screening of volunteers.

• Screening •

The initial screening should be done by someone with ability to eliminate those people whose personalities are averse to helping someone who is deeply in pain. The abrasive; the egocentric, who talk overmuch about their own loss; the neurotic, who are so caught up in their own problems that they cannot be open with another—these people should be screened out immediately. It is possible for such people to do other volunteer work that is not as sensitive, so they should not be discouraged from helping. However, the screening should select those who are sufficiently mature emotionally and sufficiently clear of their own loss experiences to be able to take on another's pain.

• Motivation •

Volunteer service is not as deeply entrenched in the United States as in the British Isles. However, with proper presentation of needs and an appeal to the proper groups, lay volunteers for grief work can be found. "Service," says Paul Maves, "is not an instrumental activity we perform for a reward, but an emotional expressive role we take because it is our nature to love as much as it is to sing."[2] Once we experience the reward of helping another, the activity itself becomes rewarding. Spiritually, we give as the writer of Psalm 23 indicates, because our cup runs over—because we have received care from others and have become aware of the grace of God in our life.

• Curriculum •

The person who is responsible for the training event needs to work out with others on the educational committee such details as the place of training, the time of training, and the texts or material to be used by the trainees. If there is to be outside leadership, those persons will need to be contacted. Finally, the course must be designed and the curricular materials obtained. In the following pages a basic training design is outlined. It should be apparent, however, that this design should be tailored to suit the training group and the situation that confronts the church or agency. It is our belief that the basic course should consist of at least eight periods, each lasting at least an hour and a half. Less time would not allow the trainer to cover the basic material, nor would the participants be able to develop sufficient group support to work through the necessary dynamic issues.

Handout For First Session

Training Exercise

1. In your notebook, describe several loss experiences. Choose losses other than death, such as moving, losing a job, leaving school, the breakup of an engagement or marriage, the loss related to aging.

   a. Describe the loss experience, answering these questions:
      Who or what was lost?
      How did the loss occur? Include time and place.
      Who was involved, or who related to you in the experience?
      How important was the loss to your life?

   b. How did you react to the loss?
      How did you feel after the loss occurred?

In your estimation, how did you handle the loss?
How did your friends/relatives think you handled the loss?
Did anything hinder you in handling the loss?
How did the experience help your growth?
How did the experience retard your growth?

2. Imagine the future loss of someone or something you hold dear, and imagine your reaction to that loss.

Visualize this experience and note your reactions either in writing or in a pencil drawing. Remain quiet before you begin, then express your feelings in your notebook or on a separate piece of paper.

Read: C. S. Lewis, *A Grief Observed* (New York: Seabury Press, 1961)

> And is there anyone at all?
> And is there anyone at all?
> I am knocking at the oaken door . . .
> And will it open
> Never now no more
> I am calling, calling to you—
> Don't you hear
> And is there anyone near?
> And does this empty silence have to be
> And is there no one there at all
> To answer me?
> I do not know the road—
> I fear to fall
> And is there anyone
> At All?[3]
>
> —*Eithne Tabor*

• First Session •

Introduction

Goal: The purpose of the session is to understand the process of normal grief and to enable the lay worker to compare his or her style of handling loss with other persons' different styles.

Objectives:
1. To provide an understanding of the normal way of handling loss.
2. To work through exercises in which counseling trainees are enabled to get in touch with their loss.
3. To help the group toward giving and receiving support while airing a loss experience.
4. To help the various workers gain insight into their own styles of handling loss.
5. To affirm each person's style as important and to discover ways for each to support his or her own style and those of others.

The Class
1. *Introduction:* What is grief? The leader centers his or her remarks on the material in chapter 2 of this book.
   15 min.
2. *Sharing Experiences of Personal Loss.* Trainees divide into small groups of 5. Each person takes 5 minutes to share the results of the first homework exercise. No discussion; only questions for clarification. 25 min.
3. *Plenary:* The leader asks each small group to share learning and feelings. These are put on newsprint.
   10 min.
4. *Visualization of Personal Loss:* In small groups of 5, each trainee shares the second homework assignment, visualizing a future grief experience. These are also put on newsprint. 30 min.
5. *Plenary:* The leader asks the recorders to place newsprint in front of total group. The leader summarizes learning, pointing out variety of styles of grieving. Emphasis is on what trainees uncovered about themselves—their losses and their styles of grieving. Secondary learning consists

of support trainees find in discussing loss in small group.   25 min.
6. *Closing:* Poem about loss is shared.
Handout for next session.

Handout for Second Session

Grief Work Skills

Three basic roles must be learned before you do actual counseling or helping work with the bereaved. These are the Expresser of feelings, the Supporter of the one who expresses feelings, and the Facilitator of interactions between two people in a helping relationship.[4]

The *Expresser* chooses subject area, speaks in regard to own feelings and perceptions, avoids talking about another's motives but focuses instead on own behavior and resultant feelings.

The Empathic Responder (Supporter) does not judge the other's feelings, uses empathy, tries to see the situation from the other's point of view, communicates acceptance and understanding, does not lead or divert with question or advice, and so on.

The Facilitator sets up the role play, provides encouragement, support, and help, gives honest feedback when the role play is over.

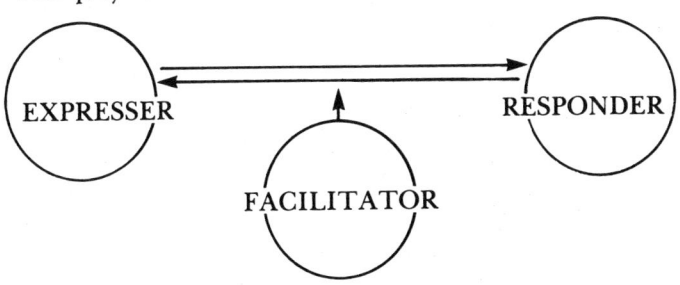

EXPRESSER ⇄ RESPONDER

FACILITATOR

In the role-play exercises we shall work out within the class, each person will be given an opportunity to play each role. The focus will be upon a loss, so that in the role play you will have an opportunity to work through the loss with a helping friend.

If you want to be the expresser in the first role play, think again about your loss experience and stay with the feelings this brings up. Put these feelings in your notebook, with just a word or two to denote the mood that is elicited.

If drawing helps, put the loss in a picture form and come to some kind of closure about the feeling.

• **Second Session** •

Learning to Listen

Goal: To teach the trainees the skills of active listening. To give them some experience in role playing these skills. To give them some feedback from group members and leader as to how they are learning these roles.

Objectives:
1. To discuss the roles of active listening in relation to the person experiencing loss.
2. To illustrate these roles in a role-play situation which the trainees may observe.
3. To give the trainees experience in role playing these skills with group members around a loss experienced by one in the group.

The Class
1. The leader discusses the principles of active listening as described on the handout. These are related to supporting one who is going through a grief experience.

The leader asks two experienced counselors to demonstrate with him/her the roles of expresser, empathic responder (supporter), and facilitator. A loss experience is selected to be the focus of the counseling. The facilitator describes the loss and sets up the role play. The role play goes on sufficiently to illustrate expressing feelings, responding to feelings, and giving feedback on the helping relationship. The group is alerted to the importance of the nonverbal, of waiting for feelings to emerge, and the difference between helpful and nonhelpful supportive statements.   45 min.
2. The leader divides the total group into triads with instructions to role play an actual loss previously described as the central focus for the role play. The person who has experienced the loss is the first facilitator, with the other two playing the expresser and supporter. Each person in the group gets a chance at each role, with honest feedback coming from the evaluator each time. Keep group moving.   30 min.
3. *Plenary:* The leader puts the learning about expressing, supporting, and evaluating on newsprint and fields questions from the group about their practice of these skills.   30 min.
4. *Conclusion:* The leader hands out the exercise for the following session on confrontation. A short period of silence, with some supportive poem being read as background, brings the session to a close.   15 min.

Handout for Third Session

Confrontation Skill Training

In the novel by Mary Gordon titled *Final Payments*, Isabelle, the main character, seeks advice from her friends

Liz and Eleanor after the death of her father. She had attended him for more than ten years during his final illness and is totally unprepared for life in the real world. Her two girlfriends must confront her directly to urge her to get a job and begin again to relate to men.[5]

Think of a time when you went to a friend with a problem and that friend "told it like it was"—that is, confronted you with your own part in the problem. Were you angry? Did it break the friendship? (Write your account of the incident.)

Did you stop and look at your part in the problem at that time? Later?

Did this style of confrontation make you any more realistic and force you from a stance of escape or withdrawal?

Now think of another time when you were grieving and may have been seeking sympathy rather than facing up to what lay ahead of you.

Answer the questions above, thinking of a friend's words to you which were confrontive, not sympathetic.

• Third Session •

Learning to Confront

Goal: The purpose is to see the nature of confrontation, and its uses in helping the griever recognize the reality of his or her situation and begin to accept the facts of loss. To give the trainees some experience in confrontation.

Objectives:
1. To allow the trainees to understand the active side of listening, confrontation.

A TRAINING MODULE

2. To give the trainees some experience in confrontation so they can distinguish it from manipulation or advice.
3. To show the place which confronting loss has in the total grief experience.

The Class

1. *Introduction:* The leader reviews the place of support, particularly in the early stages of grief. The class is made aware that there are various defenses against grieving but that a primary one is denial. The class reviews the grief cycle, and the place of confrontation at a particular stage of the grief period is demonstrated with case material. 15 min.
2. Practice a role play with two experienced persons to show how a helper confronts an expresser and, in a caring way, enables the expresser to face the problem directly. The leader will play the evaluative role and point out the differences between confrontation, manipulation, advice giving. 15 min.
3. *Group Practice:* Divide the group into triads and ask each group to work on a real loss experienced by one of the three. Have the person whose loss is being role-played as the facilitator. He or she describes the loss and starts and stops the role play. Give each person a chance at each role. 45 min.
4. *Plenary:* The leader calls the group together and discusses how the role-play experience helped the expresser through the denial of grief. If some helpers did not make helpful responses, these should be noted without blame, but by showing how the responses could be more constructive. The leader puts the learnings on newsprint, then shows what speaking the truth in love does to break the grief cycle. 15 min.
5. Form a friendship circle, closing with reading from Psalm 22 or a poem. 5 min.

Give the group The Life Line handout with instructions to bring these back next week.

Handout for Fourth Session

The Life Line

Draw a line which indicates your life line from birth to your present age, thus:

```
      10      20      30      40      50      60
L_____→
Birth
```

Note on the life line the times when you experienced significant loss, thus:

```
        Lost            Lost            Lost
        father          best            major
                        friend          job
L_____→
         12              22              45
```

Consider the most recent loss and indicate the goals you finally adopted as a way of recouping the loss.

Now prioritize those goals in terms of most important to least important.

Now look at the goals again to see whether there is any relationship between them, such as, "I must go to graduate school before I can get the next job I really want." Think about which of your goals are dreams, which have some vision but also are possible, and which are simply mundane—that is, do not represent any stretching of your capabilities.

• Fourth Session •

Learning to Motivate to Action

Goal: The purpose of the session is to enable trainees to understand the relationship between hope and goal-setting, and to engage in exercises that will increase their ability to motivate the grief-stricken person to action.

Objectives:
1. To relate hope to goal direction.
2. To understand the needs and wants of grieving persons and what inhibits them in attaining their goals.
3. To enable lay counselors to enhance grieving persons' incentives and reduce their inhibitions.
4. To show the relation between a person's goal seeking and his or her value system.

The Class
1. *Introduction.* The leader reviews the material on hope (see chapter 4). Then on newsprint, shows the relationship between goal-directed activity, intention, and inhibition (activity which blocks goal seeking) through a diagram.

I want to work. ⟶ ⟵ I need to settle the estate.

I would like to sell my house. ⟶ ⟵ I'd hate to leave this place.

　　　　I have a need to meet →← I'm afraid of strangers.
　　　　people.
　　Ask the group for additional such data from last week's
　　role play.　　　　　　　　　　　　　　　　30 min.
2. *Class Interaction:* Have trainees break into groups of 6 and work through the life line that each has prepared, spotting loss experiences but focusing on a recent loss. Have each person speak about his or her life line, the long-range goals sought at the time of the loss, how these were given some priority in goal seeking, what motivated the person in goal seeking.　　　　　　　15 min.
3. *Plenary:* Have one trainee from each group put his or her life line up before the whole group and explain what was learned about goal setting and goal seeking from the exercises. Have two experienced role players dramatize one of these situations to show the inhibitions to goal seeking and how these are intentionally worked through.　　　　　　　　　　　　　　　　30 min.
4. *Second Interaction:* Divide the class into groups of 6. Have each person show intentions and inhibitions in goal seeking, imaginatively work through the inhibitions blocking a short-range goal, and report this to the group.　　　　　　　　　　　　　　　　　15 min.
5. *Second Plenary:* Put class learning about goal seeking and motivation on newsprint. The leader will show how goal setting and prioritizing of goals demonstrate the value system of the individual.　　　　　　　　　15 min.

Conclusion

　　Read from Frankl, or give it as a handout, as each trainee meditates on what she or he values most at this point in life.
　　Excerpt from Viktor E. Frankl, *From Death-Camp to Existentialism:*

> An active life serves the purpose of giving man the opportunity to realize values in creative work, while a passive life of enjoyment affords him the opportunity to obtain fulfillment in

experiencing beauty, art, or nature. But there is also purpose in that life which is almost barren of both creation and enjoyment and which admits of but one possibility of high moral behavior: namely, in man's attitude to his existence, an existence restricted by external forces. A creative life and a life of enjoyment are banned to him. But not only creativeness and enjoyment are meaningful. If there is a meaning in life at all, then there must be a meaning in suffering. Suffering is an ineradicable part of life, even as fate and death. Without suffering and death human life cannot be complete.

The way in which a man accepts his fate and all the suffering it entails, the way in which he takes up his cross, gives him ample opportunity—even under the most difficult circumstances—to add a deeper meaning to his life. It may remain brave, dignified and unselfish. Or in the bitter fight for self-preservation he may forget his human dignity and become no more than an animal. Here lies the chance for a man either to make use of or to forgo the opportunities of attaining the moral values that a difficult situation may afford him. And this decides whether he is worthy of his sufferings or not.[6]

Handout for Fifth Session

Life Review Exercise

Return to your life line which you drew last week. Work with the current place in your life and assess just where you are in overcoming loss.

```
                              Current Loss
       10      20      30      40      50      60
|_____→
Birth                 ------→
              (Events that led up to loss)
```

What events led up to the loss experience? List these.

What was the state of your relationship with significant people in your life at the time?

What was your state of health? Did you have any long period when you were worn out from your work, or missed sleep worrying about your situation?

Did you seek out anyone to talk with about your situation, or did you keep it to yourself?

Did you at that time have a significant network of persons whom you felt cared about you, and if so, who were they?

Was your faith of any help to you, or did you feel that God had turned his back on you, that you were alone in your suffering? Be perfectly frank about this.

Now show this in a diagram. Example:

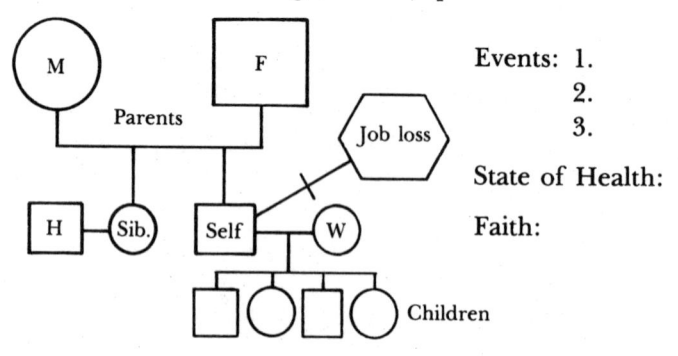

```
   M         F                    Events: 1.
      Parents                             2.
                    Job loss              3.
  H — Sib.  Self — W             State of Health:
         Children                 Faith:
```

• **Fifth Session** •

*Bringing the Grieving to Honest Self-Evaluation
and New Relationships*

Goal: The purpose of the session is to teach the lay counselor to bring the grieving to honest self-evaluation and enable them to form new relationships with others.

Objectives:
1. To help the bereaved move beyond abnormal guilt and self-blame in relation to loss.
2. To help the bereaved evaluate themselves as accepted and affirmed.
3. To move the bereaved toward meaningful group activities.
4. To help the bereaved relate to new acquaintances and friends.

The Class
1. *Introduction:* The leader discusses life review as a process (see chapter 4). The leader uses his or her own example, and with life review shows how a major loss was overcome. The example is diagrammed on newsprint as the trainees have been instructed to do for the lesson. 30 min.
2. *Group Work:* The class is divided into groups of 6, with the life review charts as a basis of discussion. Each person spends 5 minutes showing the life review which went on at the time of loss, the decisions made, and the resources found to take up life anew. Other group members search for moments of self-acceptance in the discussion.
30 min.
3. *Plenary:* The leader asks for learning from the life review from each group, with focus on self-acceptance and self-affirmation. Then the leader discusses own life review, showing how he or she moved into new situations following the loss, emphasizing the forming of new friendships. 25 min.
4. *Group Work:* The class breaks up into triads for role play of one such loss. The three roles of expresser,

empathizer, and facilitator are role-played. The emphasis should be on enabling the bereaved to reach out in friendship toward one other person in his or her life. Defenses against doing this are not bulldozed but dealt with firmly yet supportively. The facilitator gives feedback before the role play shifts. Each person gets a chance to play the bereaved, the counselor, and the evaluator. 25 min.
5. *Conclusion:* The leader summarizes the meaningfulness of seeing oneself in relation to the whole of one's life journey. He or she also affirms each person's presentation and shows the value of self-acceptance. The group ends with a friendship circle, affirming the friends made in this group. The Ritual Exercise handout is given to each trainee. 10 min.

Handout for Sixth Session

Ritual Exercise

Ritual is older than language, say anthropologists. It is made up of movement and drama centering around the elementary experiences of one's existence. Tribes and families built ritual into their experiences of birth, coming of age, marriage, and death. It is around the dying experience that we shall ritualize in this coming week.

Think of the rites which surround death in your family and ethnic group. Make a list of these.

Separate the rites that are memorials to the departed from those that are meant to comfort and sustain the living.

In *Last Letter to the Pebble People,* the author tells about a ritual she and her family developed. Each evening at 5:00 P.M. they dropped a pebble into a fountain and engaged in a meditation centering on Aldie, who was terminally ill with cancer. Aldie died, but with the support of his family and friends.[7] Do you have any private experience which has sustained you during the loss of a friend or relative? Write it in your notebook.

• **Sixth Session** •

Acknowledging the Spiritual Needs of the Bereaved

Goal: The purpose of this lesson is to discuss the spiritual needs of each trainee so as to help members of the group become more aware of their similarities and differences. It is also to show how ritual helps people express their cry for meaning and put their lives in the context of the generations. Despite different spiritual backgrounds, this session should bind trainees closer together in their quest for meaning.

Objectives:
1. To examine the cry for meaning at the time of death and loss.
2. To hear the variety of ways people handle death in Jewish, Roman Catholic, Protestant, and secular settings.
3. To understand the place of ritual in these various contexts of dying and loss.
4. To see the spiritual needs of families in their particular family systems.

The Class
1. If the teacher is a clergyperson, two others from different faith groups should be invited to discuss the spiritual needs of the bereaved. If the leader is a lay person, clergy from the three faith groups should be invited. They should be asked not to deliver a sermon, but to speak out of their pastoral experiences at the time

of the death of a significant person. They should tell what they have learned from church people and from nonchurch people at the time of loss. 30 min.
2. *Group Activity:* The class is divided into groups of 6, with the clergy asked to join as resource people. The group members should tell about the rites that are a part of their faith or ethnic group. They should share also, if they desire, the private rites they have devised to help them through a period of grief. Each clergyperson listens and remarks on the spiritual needs these rites address, and how the transcendent mystery of life and death is faced through ritual. 45 min.
3. *Plenary:* The whole group discusses the learnings, with the leader putting the insights on newsprint. The group closes with a friendship circle. The leader lifts the arms of the participants in praise and, after a 3-minute silence, repeats one sentence affirming God as the Ruler of life and death. 30 min.

Handout for Seventh Session

Support Groups

Carl Rogers has written:

> I feel that risk-taking is one of the many things I myself have learned from experience in encounter groups. Though I do not always live up to it, I have learned that there is basically nothing to be afraid of. When I present myself as I *am,* when I can come forth nondefensively, without armor, just me—when I can accept the fact that I have many deficiencies and faults, make many mistakes, and am often ignorant where I should be knowledgeable, often prejudiced when I should be open-minded, often have feelings which are not justified by the circumstances—then I can be much more real. And when I can

come out wearing no armor, making no effort to be different from what I am, I learn much more—even from criticism and hostility—and am much more relaxed and get much closer to people. . . .

This willingness to take the risk of being one's inner self is certainly one of the steps toward relieving the loneliness that exists in each one of us and putting us in genuine touch with other human beings.[8]

It is not enough to turn inward toward spiritual sources for strength and guidance; one needs to turn outward toward individuals and groups that can be of help. List organizations you know of that offer support groups.

List the key persons who lead such groups, or who could be asked to lead such groups.

List the ways this class has been a support for you in the past few weeks.

• Seventh Session •

Motivating the Bereaved to Join Support Groups

Goal: The purpose of the session is to enable trainees to motivate the bereaved to join support groups. The leader will utilize the class as an example of a support group and have it reflect on the value of group activity.

Objectives:
1. To understand the need of the bereaved for the support of others who have experienced loss.
2. To reflect on the responses of group members to the supportive, confronting, and enabling help of others.

3. To help the group become aware of where such groups may exist or where they should be organized.
4. To motivate grievers to join such support groups.

The Class

1. The leader will summarize the grief cycle which the grief counselors have worked through. The grief worker needs to understand that he or she does not work alone but that support groups offer continuing help over the first year of bereavement. The leader asks the members to reflect on how the training group has helped them confront their need for stimulation, support, and motivation to act. These insights are put before the class on newsprint. The leader asks members to find 5 others with whom they are most compatible and form a support group. The leader is sensitive to the shy people who are slow in their choice and helps them form the final group. 30 min.
2. Each support group is asked to reflect on the losses originally listed in the first session. Each member then speaks of how particular members in the group have helped them:
    a) in a supportive way.
    b) in a confrontive way
    c) in helping to relate again to others
    d) in motivating to activity 30 min.
3. *Plenary:* The recorder puts the learnings on newsprint and brings them back to the total group where they are posted. The leader speaks of the value of having those who have lost someone in death work with other bereaved for the first year after the loss. The question is then raised as to whether such groups are available.
   35 min.
4. *Collation of Information:* The leader collects information from the total group about grief-recovery groups in the area. If there is a paucity of such groups, the leader

discusses the availability of leaders, meeting places, and organizational details necessary to start such groups. Churches, hospices, Ys, lodges, granges, even vacant rooms or homes can be considered. Before the evening is over, several persons should be given responsibility to follow up suggestions about finding or organizing such groups. 30 min.
5. *Conclusion:* Group evaluation form is given out to be returned at last session. Finding and Making Referrals handout is distributed.

Group Evaluation

(Reproduce for each member of group to respond in writing.)

1. What met your expectations?
   What did not meet your expectations?
2. Do you think you are now ready to do bereavement counseling?
3. If not, explain where you think you need more training.
4. Would you recommend the course to a friend? If yes, why? If no, why not?
5. What would you change in the format of the course to improve it?

Handout for Eighth Session

Finding and Making Referrals

The two types of bereaved with whom you will work are those who can handle their grief with supportive counseling, and those for whom a referral to professional psychotherapeutic help is needed. The purpose of this exercise is to begin to make you aware of the difference between the normally grieved and the severely grieved.

From your learning so far, on the grief cycle shown below—shock-disorganization-reorganization—list the signs of severe grief.

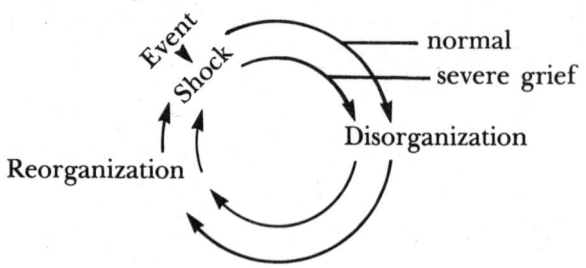

```
         Event
            ↓              ——— normal
         Shock             ——— severe grief
                    ↘
   ↑↑                    Disorganization
                    ↙
Reorganization
         ↙
```

Have you ever been in the presence of severe grief? If so, how did it make you feel?

What do you think is the usual period for moving from disorganization to reorganization? Think of this in terms of a loss you have suffered.

Granted that you now have some skills in supporting, confronting, and enabling a griever to point outward toward the world, what would you do if you found these skills were not working?

You have one person, the teacher of your course, to whom you can turn. Do you feel that you could talk frankly about a grief-stricken person who appears depressed, suicidal, or to be drifting apathetically without purpose? If the answer is yes, do you think you could still follow this person in care after you obtain professional help?

• Eighth Session •

Bringing the Severely Bereaved to Professional Help

Goal: The purpose of this session is to enable the trainee to distinguish the severely bereaved from one going through normal grief; it will also enable the trainee to make a referral and to continue supportive help to the grieving person after referral.

Objectives:
1. To draw on the trainee's experience with his or her own grief or with another's grief so as to be able to understand the difference between normal grief and severe grief.
2. To acquaint the trainees with a professional who treats the severely bereaved.
3. To make the trainees aware of those in the community available to help the severely bereaved individual and/or family.
4. To show the trainees their caretaking is not over, once a referral is made.

The Class
1. The leader (if not a professional care-giver) will invite a professional—psychiatrist, psychologist, social worker, or trained pastoral counselor—to discuss the difference between normal and severe grief. The grief wheel should be used to show how normal grief may expand to severe grief if the normal process through grieving is aborted or stuck. The professional should speak the layperson's language and draw illustrations from his or her work experience to enliven the presentation. Family systems with the emotional shock wave effect of loss should be illustrated. Time for questions should be allowed.

   45 min.
2. *Group Practice:* The class should divide into triads with the expresser, counselor, and facilitator roles assigned. If each triad cannot think of a severe case to work with, the leader or professional care-giver should have several such cases available in written form to role play. These should come out of their experience and be sufficiently disguised so that no one in the group can recognize the cases. Role play three times, with each person role

playing a referral, and the evaluator waiting until the role play is finished to give feedback. Problems or questions should be brought back to the plenary.

30 min.

3. *Final Plenary:* The leader handles the final questions about referral with help from the professional caregiver. The group is told that there will be a follow-up interview with each trainee and that continuing supervision will be made available as they begin their supportive care-giving.
4. *Conclusion:* The final evaluation of the group sessions are handed in. Each trainee is asked to say in one sentence what the training experience has meant to him or her. The leader asks the group to form a friendship circle to sing a closing song—*Amazing Grace, Blest Be the Tie That Binds,* or another group-binding song. 15 min.

Continued Supervision of the Lay Grief Worker

The authors assume that the leader of the grief work training is a supervisor with some accrediting group such as ACPE, AAPC, AASW, APA, or another. If this is not so, then the leader should secure such a person or persons to carry out the continuing supervision of the trainees. Ongoing supervision should be seen as a necessity for the lay grief counselor. The lay workers should have understood through the final session that they can get beyond their competency, that they can lose motivation, or simply go stale if their work does not come under review by a professional counselor.

What do we mean by supervision?

The various groups define supervision in different ways, but the lay workers should understand that supervision has a close relationship with good teaching. Whereas they have been learning with others, with role play as the primary teaching medium, now they will be actually calling on the bereaved. The content, context, and dynamics of the call now become the focus for learning.

The supervisor and care-giver or givers should have a definite time and place for meeting. This can be weekly, bi-weekly, but surely no less often than once a month, depending upon the arrangement each can work out. The place can be a hospice, a church, an agency, or school. The trainer may see only one trainee for a supervisory hour, or as many as four at a time. Each person should have adequate time to discuss his or her counseling work; otherwise the experience will lack the depth and intensity necessary for continued learning. We recommend group supervision because of the group's *supportive* help.

The materials for supervision are made available through the lay counselor's
—memory of the client contact
—process notes
—a verbatim account
—audio or video tape-recording.

The latter method, although the most expensive, gives the most reliable feedback of the counseling session. The supervisory process can be outlined as follows:

1. The care-giver *recalls* contact with the griefstricken. The supervisor questions the counselor to help fill in gaps in the description of what led up to the loss, current behavior, and attempts of the griefstricken to reorder his or her life.

2. *Review* the flow of the helper's responses in relation to the grieving person's expression of where he or she is. The supervisor is sensitive to the stage and style of grief and to the counselor's helpful and unhelpful responses.
3. *Anticipate* the next stage of grief. The supervisor and counselor attempt to understand whether the griever is making progress, is stuck, or is regressing, so as to decide the proper strategy to follow in counseling.
4. *Strategize* the grief counselor's helping responses. What will the counselor's response be to the movement, inertia, or regression of the griever? How can he or she be of most help to the bereaved next time?
5. *Evaluate* the grief counselor's overall stance and particular interventions in relation to a style or method. The supervisor takes time to reinforce the counselor's growth and to support change where advisable.

Continuing Education for the Lay Grief Worker

Although the initial training gives the grief counselors a start, and although continuing supervision keeps them going, continuing education is a necessity. Bereavement work can drain a counselor of emotional resources more readily than any other kind of helping. When symptoms of burnout appear, when loss strikes a grief worker and it is necessary to attend to his or her own grief, or when another crisis happens which interferes with caring, he or she should take a leave from the caring activity. Continuing education will help to replenish resources and so, in particular, will association with people who have broad interests and a lively sense of living. If one is a volunteer, some activity which puts one in touch with living, growing, and dynamic activity should be sought out. Above all, the grief worker should relate to a religious community, a group of people with a purpose and a weekly ritual which sustains them over the days and months. A communion with the ground of meaning and hope beyond oneself and beyond the generations will sustain one when all else fails.

Notes

1. Howard Thurman, *Meditations of the Heart* (New York: Harper & Row, 1953), pp. 212-13.
2. Eithne Tabor, from *The Cliff's Edge: Songs of a Psychotic* (London: Sheed & Ward Ltd., 1951). Reprinted by permission.
3. Paul Maves, *Older Volunteers in Church and Community* (Valley Forge, Pa.: Judson Press, 1981).
4. Bernard Guerney, *Relationship Enhancement* (San Francisco: Jossey-Bass, 1977).
5. Mary Gordon, *Final Payments* (New York: Random House, 1978).
6. Viktor E. Frankl, *From Death-Camp to Existentialism* (Boston: Beacon Press, 1959), pp. 66-67.
7. Virginia H. Hine, *Last Letter to the Pebble People* (Santa Cruz, Calif.: Unity Press, 1979).
8. Carl Rogers, *Carl Rogers on Encounter Groups* (New York: Harper & Row, 1970), pp. 113-14.

EIGHT

Outline of a Death and Dying Seminar

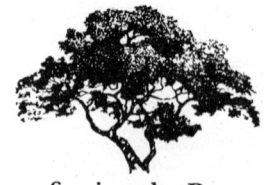

When our small group first gathered to discuss our concern for providing better care for dying persons and their families, we were concerned primarily as professionals. But as we continued to talk for several months about death, dying, and bereavement it became clear that we were not just professionally, but personally involved. One evening as we met in the Dobihal living room we were struggling to arrive at a "philosophy" that would undergird hospice care.

The statement couldn't be too theological, for we were a very mixed religious group—humanist, Protestant, Jewish, Roman Catholic, perplexed. But we were a serious group, concerned for others, concerned for ourselves, open about differences, and surprised sometimes by similarities. We had shared enough of our stories in various ways to know that all of us, as human beings, had experienced life, death, bereavement. We didn't approach the subject as objective clinicians or care-givers. We were participants in a life process, wanting to express in our philosophy our feeling of being partners with others in the journey of life and death. In April of 1971, a tentative statement was drafted:

> The philosophy of the projected Hospice evolves from our personal experiences with life and death and particularly our shared experiences over this past year—experiences with patients whose remaining life time has been short and with their families, professionals, and all others close to the patient.
>
> Our work during this exploratory period leads us to appreciate the therapeutic force made available to patients and their families when the individuals providing care are drawn together and motivated by a deep-seated reverence for human life and its inherent struggles during crises.
>
> The professional and scientific knowledge of nursing and medicine, combined with this reverence for life and its spirit, serves to help the staff understand the experiences of the patient and family and to relieve their distress. We find that this type of care increases the capacity of the patient and family to live through this period with meaning and dignity. It is important to discover the patient's and family's life-style so that we can adapt to them and help them include this experience of

dying and bereavement in their life, in their own way. The patient and family, therefore, assume active roles in the decision making processes. They also become teachers for other patients and families and for staff members seeking to be more understanding and helpful during this moment of crisis in life experience. Thus the work of the Hospice is shared among patients, families, and staff, all cooperating in the caring task.

Persons who help terminally ill patients round out their lives expend tremendous energy; this needs replenishing. Patients and families help with this replenishment, but since they come and go there is need to recognize the importance of the ongoing relations of the Hospice workers to one another. This is the Hospice "family" which welcomes those in need, serves them and helps them on their way. This "family," in its openness and concern for all members, is what sustains. It is necessary for all in the Hospice to be both strong and weak, giver and receiver, and to be strengthened by bonds between people and not only by one's internal resources.

Our philosophy cannot be a creed and yet our explorations and growing bonds often cause us to say, "We believe." We believe in honoring the creed and philosophy of every man. We believe in the dignity of personhood—patients, families, workers—and will nurture a spirit of respect for every person. We believe in the importance of feelings, in the fact that there are differences between people to be creatively shared, in love which can be experienced between people and will support them. Some say "We believe in God" in different ways, but important in that our daily work reflects a purpose that is beyond us and is moving us.

This philosophy cannot be concluded in words, for it is one to be tested in action, to remain open to the learning that will come from our relationships with each other, and to be creatively changed and added to. Our serving, our teaching, our research, all will add to our knowledge and may change our philosophy. But we are growing as a group and perhaps that will be a most important source of further change—the creativity that will come from our group mind, greater than any of our single minds, or from what we could call our group spirit.

This statement of an early group, thinking about death, dying, bereavement, established a base upon which to found their ministry. It was open-ended, recognizing that time and experience would bring change and, we hoped, positive refinements. It still contains many true principles to be considered by persons who seek to move forward, create their own philosophy statements, and expand their view of life to include death.

Following are suggestions for a training unit or educational program that will help you bring death and dying back into life. You will become the writers of a new chapter of life that will give individuals, families, congregations new options for including death as part of life. I am excited, since I do not know what those options will be—I believe God is working in the world and you will work with our creator in ways that are still a mystery. I will make suggestions and have faith that your beginning will bear new fruit.

Beginnings

Where to begin?—a vital first question and one that will be answered differently by different pastors and parishes. Some will be thinking seriously about this field of ministry for the very first time. Some pastors may have been concerned about these issues, but their parishioners may be only dimly aware, not knowing exactly where they fit in this ministry. Other churches may be very knowledgeable of a hospice program, may be contributing to it financially, may have members as volunteers or on the staff, and so possess considerable awareness of a program of terminal care. Other churches may have discussed and made statements on such segments of the topic as the Christian funeral, the living will.

Take stock of where your church is with reference to death, dying, and bereavement issues. That is the only place to begin. Who should do that? Not just the pastor! . . . nor the staff if it is a large church! These are concerns of all the people of the parish. Somehow the church community needs to be involved in the process of reflection, decision making, and any program planning that appears necessary.

In some churches the community may be represented by an already existing group: a church committee; the board of deacons, or vestry, or council on ministries; an educational group. However, there are two dangers if this type of group assumes the task.

Danger No. 1: *Death, dying, and bereavement is a topic that involves all of us in anxiety.* That is one of the reasons we avoid the subject and its implications for us. An existing group will have a number of responsibilities and thus be able to escape to another task if the anxiety level begins to rise. Usually this does not happen by conscious choice. After a sudden burst of enthusiasm the group gets very busy with all its other important responsibilities, and sometime later wonders what happened to those issues of "dying." They had died, been buried in other work, and life had gone on. That's a very familiar process, parallel to the death of an individual—a flurry of concern, then the funeral, and then life goes on—except for the bereaved. If an existing group is chosen for this task, there will be some who will mourn the project's loss if the danger I have described does occur. Those mourners will bring the group back to the issue and perhaps should become a nucleus to carry the task further.

Danger No. 2: *Death, dying, and bereavement is a topic that involves all of us in anxiety.* This second reason is the same as the first. Many people in the congregation have attitudes and ideas about existing groups in the church structure. Those groups are made up of people "I like" or "I don't like" or "I know" or "I don't know." Oh, that group has the job of running the church, or taking care of the property, or bearing the responsibility for the budget and business, or conducting the educational programs, or whatever.

No matter which existing group assumes the task, the people of the congregation who have other responsibilities on other groups, and those who may only attend worship, will be able to escape the anxiety of the topic (if they even know it is being thought about) by saying, "I'm glad somebody else is doing that!" Then they can ignore it peacefully, with the knowledge that somebody else is doing something important.

To avoid these dangers the pastor and one of the

policy-making groups of the church may discuss and decide that indeed it is important for the entire church community to consider the variety of issues involved in death, dying, and bereavement. They may then choose a few of themselves to gather a group (now very popularly called a task force) to consider this topic in view of their specific congregation. This would be a new group, with one task, and it would allow for announcements in the bulletin and newsletter, statements from the pulpit, invitations for people with experience and expertise to join and interested volunteers to step forward from the congregation.

Again, churches have different forms and different styles. It may be that your church is well acquainted with task forces. Perhaps your style is that one person would stand up on Sunday morning, state an interest in death, dying, and bereavement, and invite others who are interested to come to the altar rail after the service and form a task force on the topic. Fine. The method for beginning will vary. But keep in mind a few basic facts:

1. The topic/issue/project does arouse anxiety which can surface as denial of its importance, resistance to its being considered, or acceptance and then avoidance of the task.
2. The pastor may or may not be the key person in this project but his or her support and participation will be helpful in many ways.
3. Issues of life and death are important to everyone in the community of the church. All will not be involved, will not be touched in the same way, but the issues involve all.

4. Persons who are motivated because of their personal experience with this topic are as important as those motivated by their professional encounters and expertise (doctors, nurses, social workers, clergy). When both types of individuals come together, it can work well for the whole congregation.

Tasks/Projects/What Needs to Happen

These will vary so much in the different gatherings of people we call congregations that I will only give a few general areas the tasks probably need to include. I will outline one program which I hope will be adaptable to specific congregations.

Consciousness raising has become a popular term in recent years in connection with such varied life topics as civil rights, energy, the third world, feminism, and the topic of this book—death, dying, and bereavement. The main thrust of a local church program should be toward consciousness raising. It should move, however, from being conscious *about* the topic to being more personally involved with it individually and corporately as the church. Our consciousness should include:
1. Our shared experiences and feelings about death, dying, and bereavement.
2. Our increased awareness of the perceptions that persons who have lived through the experience can share with us.
3. Knowledge about the options for terminal care that are or are not yet available to us.

4. Creative possibilities for the life of the congregation, particularly in meeting the essential aloneness of these experiences through support.
5. Creative support of our faith.

In your congregation you may need to focus on one, three, or all five of those areas. Since you know your own situation best you may also wish to add six, seven, and eight. Good!—you do need to think in specifics arising out of your unique situation. I will now briefly outline a program that would be one way to follow through on the five areas I have listed.

First, you have gathered together that small group of persons who have committed themselves to discussing the topic. They then plan to introduce a program of a minimum of five two-hour sessions to the congregation. They will ask people to commit a minimum of ten hours to one another for the purpose of Reflecting on Death, Dying, and Bereavement. (I leave a better program title to your creative imagination.) They also limit the number of people who can be involved in this program to twenty.

Suggestions:
1. Some individual, some pair (preferably male and female who work well together), or some small group (those who work exceptionally well together) needs to be in charge—people who are comfortable with the subject, comfortable working with small groups and with a larger group (12 or more), and who can listen and adapt to the results of discussion.
2. The leader(s) need to be responsive to the fact

that they don't know what will be presented and are confident that the Spirit will lead them. A degree of humility and some trust in their brothers and sisters helps.
3. It is important to adhere to the beginning and ending time for each session. However, you have several sessions, so all the work does not have to be accomplished in the first one. Stick to the topic, modify times between the beginning and end (2, 2 1/2, or 3 hours—agreed on ahead of time), and be very careful to note the questions or issues left for future sessions.
4. Stress the importance of the assignments and of the commitment of each person to every other member of the group. Ask participants to call the leader(s) if they must be absent so that the whole group will know who is missing, and why.

• First Session •

Me—and Death, Dying, and Bereavement

Purpose:
1. To help congregational members discuss their feelings about death, dying, and bereavement with one another.
2. To identify the fears, concerns, and hopes that are most common in this group of individuals.
3. To help family members identify the similarities and differences in their views, for further discussion.

Method:
1. Give each person 20 to 30 minutes to answer these

questions. (All suggested time limits are only guides. The leader should observe the group and decide on time limits based on the activity within the group.)

Now this is an exercise that you will not in your real life be able to perform, but *if* you could:
- a. How would you choose to die? When would that be? (Two answers are required.)
- b. How would you choose *not* to die? When would you *not* want to die? (Two answers.)
- c. Think of the person to whom you are closest. Which one would you choose to die first—you or the other person? Why? (Two answers.) 20 to 30 min.

2. Ask the individuals to gather in groups of four or five to share their answers. You may want husbands and wives to be together, but I would recommend they be in different groups. Try to have some men and some women in each group—they look at things differently. Also, try to mix the ages. 30 min.

3. Bring the whole group together and start getting input from each group—one at a time—with questions like:

    Were there any surprises?
    Did some of you agree?
    Were there different opinions?

    The leader should write down key words or phrases about each of the questions on newsprint. These words and phrases can be put up each time the group meets, to show where you began.

    There will be a repetition of themes as you gather this information:

    I don't want to be a burden!
    I want to die quickly! in my sleep!
    I want to have time to say goodbye but not too much time!

I want to die after I'm 80 if I still have all my faculties!
I want to still be enjoying life when I die!
I don't want to be in a lot of pain!
I don't want to burn to death!
I'm ready to die any time now!
I don't want to die until my children are grown!
I want to die first because selfishly I don't think I could bear the grief!
I think my spouse should die first because I want to save him/her the pain!
I should die first because the children are young and need their mother!
I should die first because the children are young and need their father to provide security. 30 min.

If you did not take a coffee/tea break between sections 2 and 3, you need one now—if your group contains 15 to 20 people.

4. Now the group returns to reflect on their responses written on the newsprint.

   I want to die quickly in my sleep.—What does that do to the bereaved?
   I want to have time to say goodbye.—How would you do that?
   I don't want to be a burden.—Is it harder to receive than to give?
   I want to die first. . . . I think my spouse should die first.—What do we each give? What are our shared strengths?

5. Close with a time of silence, prayer, or perhaps a hymn such as "Blest Be the Tie That Binds."

Assignment:
1. The group is divided in half and each person is given the

name of another person. They know who they are—they are not secret pals—and they agree to have a phone conversation to exchange reflections on the session. Husbands and wives can pair with each other and commit themselves to one conversation on the topic during the week.
2. Individuals are to jot down losses they remember in their life, and how they coped with them. Examples: going to school the first day, the pet that died, not making the team, getting married, moving, a parent died, graduating, and such.

• **Second Session** •

My Losses—My Learnings from Life

Purpose:
1. To help congregational members share the losses they have experienced and the way they coped with those losses.
2. To help identify losses in which grief was not recognized.
3. To help identify losses when they were "protected" from their grief.
4. To help identify concerns of "How do we help each other?"

Method:
1. Give each person one or two pieces of newsprint and a magic marker, and ask them to take a few minutes to write down, perhaps abbreviated, the losses they made notes about during the week. This really was an assignment and this exercise demonstrates that assignments are to be taken seriously. The people who thought

you were kidding can do it on the spot and not be embarrassed.
2. The group can take time to walk around and look at the pieces of newsprint, which have been put up on the wall.
3. Reflect together on the support people those losses suggest were needed at various times in your lives.
   a. Are there childhood times your church school staff needs to be aware of?
   b. Are there adolescent times for your junior and senior high school advisors to think about?
   c. What about pastoral issues when couples are planning to marry—are they giving up some freedom? What about times when babies are born and baptized—do they also claim some of your freedom?
   d. What about job changes, moving—how do you celebrate endings, new beginnings?
   e. What about retirement—is life only work?
4. That discussion should take you at least half way through the session. If it becomes very involved, it may take the whole session. You see why the leadership must be flexible. If it looks as though it will take the whole session, you may have to ask the group if it will meet for six rather than five sessions.
5. If you have completed this part of the session in an hour, show the film *Whose Life Is It Anyway?* This is a moving film about a disabled person who is deciding whether his life should continue.
6. Provide time for discussion. The film should not be shown without time afterward for silence, reflection, feeling your response. Discuss and be prepared for different points of view. It really helps people think about the question "Whose life is it?" The answer is—mine. What does that mean?
7. A closing of silence and sentence prayers.

Assignment:
1. This type of series, for people who become serious about it, necessitates some reading, which may be assigned at the beginning and read during the five weeks. For this session Norman Cousin's book *Anatomy of an Illness* or Stewart Alsop's *Stay of Execution* would be pertinent. Others helpful to the series are Kübler-Ross, *On Death and Dying* or *Death: The Final Stage of Growth;* Sandol Stoddard, *The Hospice Movement: A Better Way of Caring for the Dying.* All books and films mentioned are noted in the bibliography. (With due humility, the chapters in this book might also be helpful as text.)
2. Think about: Deaths I have experienced. . . . their pains, problems, questions.

• Third Session •

Bereavement—Its Pain

Purpose:

1. To help the members to see that death can come at any time—not only at four score and ten.
2. To consider the response to the death of a child or young person.
3. To see that the death of a dreamed-for future goes on and on, unlike the death after a lifetime which has been lived and can be remembered.
4. To emphasize the importance of the now, the present of life.

Method:

1. Show the film *When a Child Dies.* (The leader(s) need to preview it and be well prepared to lead the discussion.)

2. If possible, have a member of The Compassionate Friends present to discuss the film with you and/or share their story of how this group has helped them to cope with such a loss.

Assignment:
Read Bradford Smith's *Dear Gift of Life* and meditate on its meaning for your life.

• Fourth Session •

Options for Dying

Purpose:
1. To begin conversations with one another about the hospice program of care.
2. To reflect on whether this option exists in your community for you and others in the congregation.
3. To reflect on whether this is an option you personally want—not all persons do.

Method:
Build this whole session around the film *As Long As There Is Life*, produced by The Connecticut Hospice, Inc., and The Hospice Institute for Education, Training, and Research. There is an excellent discussion guide prepared for use with this film. You won't be able to use all its suggestions in one showing. It was designed for programs like this and for groups seriously planning a hospice program. The latter use it in multiple showings.
1. The person(s) or couple leading this session should carefully study the discussion guide and preview the film.

2. For this evening, and probably for all evenings, some refreshments should be available for break times, at the close, or during the program, as appropriate.
3. Briefly introduce and then show this film about a real family. There is a written transcription of the dialogue which you can request when you order the film. This helps the leaders and groups to "hear" accurately and to recall.
4. After you have viewed the film leave the lights off for a few minutes and then suggest that maybe now is the time for a refreshment break. Most people find this a very moving film and don't want to plunge right into discussion.
5. During the discussion, use those portions of the guide you have selected as most important for your group.
6. Remember your purposes for this session:

   The hospice program of care—mainly home care, patient and family care.

   Is hospice care available for you in your community?
   Is it something you personally want?

Assignment:

The following assignments are based on the assumption that the next session is your last. So you need to terminate and look to the future.

1. Reflect on the four sessions and what they have meant to you—learning about the topic, about yourself, about others in the group.
2. Are there things you have done during this series or that you now need to do?
   a. Prepare a will? . . . revise it?
   b. Prepare a living will and discuss it with the necessary people?

c. Think of ways your faith, your congregation, your pastor can support you in this life journey.
3. Are there thoughts of how these topics can be helpfully considered in the life of the church?
   a. In worship and preaching?
   b. In the educational program?
   c. Should the series be repeated sometime for others?
   d. Do you have a guide on the Christian funeral specifically for your church?
   e. Do you need a bereavement team? (chapter 7)
   f. Do you need to work toward making the hospice program of care an available option for yourself and other church members?

• Fifth Session •

Ending and Beginnings

Purpose:

To leave one another and give birth to the future.

Method:

1. Leader(s) should be sure all the various newsprint material produced by the group is on display.
2. Give participants some time to be silent, read, remember. (Perhaps a record can be playing some of the great church music dealing with death and resurrection.)
3. Divide into smaller groups of four or five and share the three most important discoveries each has made during the series. How do these affect their life with one another, as well as individually?

4. The small groups or the whole group now share ideas as to how they see this topic being integrated into the life of the church.
5. Conclude with worship, perhaps Eucharist/Communion, and refreshments. This whole session might be developed around a potluck meal, discussions, worship, and dessert.

Assignment:

Go forth and put your learning, your plans, into practice.

I did not suggest that "experts" or resource people be used in this series. It is not designed to present a great deal of factual data about the topic, but to allow the people of the church to share their experiences with one another. The most important need is for a couple or leader(s) who are familiar with group work and can help people share.

The suggested series could hardly be shortened. It could be lengthened by spending more time on bereavement or on the hospice segment. A fine session could be developed on death and the arts, including the use of literature, poetry, music, and paintings. Also, you may want more time to think of your church programming. The fifth session, however, will move you back into your regular church structure—into worship, education, and the corporate life of the church as a supporting community. Perhaps your church will want to develop a bereavement team. Then further education will be needed as described in chapter 7.

I hope that the series, whether extending over five

weeks or carried out on a planning retreat or at a summer camp, will be helpful to the individuals involved, who will have shared rather intimate thoughts, feelings, and concerns. Also, I hope the topic of death, dying, and bereavement will have been a lively one, life-enriching for individuals and for the church.

NINE

Developing a Grief Support Group

by Dora Elaine Tiller

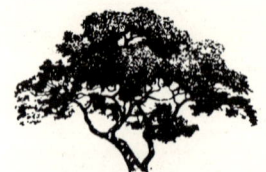

Grief is an isolating experience; persons who are grieving are often depressed, angry, lonely, sad, unsure of themselves and their future. These feelings are hard to share because of the deep internal sense that they are not acceptable to others: "Either I as a grieving person must hide these feelings and pretend, or I must withdraw and isolate myself." Coupled with this attitude are the signals the griever is receiving from associates. Most of us are not very good at listening to negative feelings, so well-intentioned neighbors, friends, and family frequently attempt to console the griever with such platitudes as, "It's time to get over it," "At least he's not suffering anymore," "You have to keep busy." All these sound to the griever like "Come on already, I can't take your being upset anymore." Thus in my job as grief counselor, I listen to many grieving persons who tell me it's a lonely existence because when they are with most persons, they must pretend they are just fine. Besides their loss and grief, they have the added burden of protecting others from feeling the pain they are feeling. Churches are beginning to reach out to persons who are grieving because of the death of a friend or family member by developing grief support groups. As there is power "in community" within the church in general, there is power "in community" for those who have suffered the death of a loved one.

When persons who are grieving come together in a support group, they are given the opportunity to air their feelings and to learn that, indeed, these feelings are also a part of others' grief: "What a relief to be accepted as a grieving person by five to ten other persons, and what a relief to learn that my feelings are not unique and ridiculous. What a relief to find I'm not going crazy—if others share these feelings, they're validated and okay; therefore, I am okay."

Also in this group experience of shared grief there is the sense that "I will be able to grow through this experience." The day one group member is very low, other members will feel up; thus they carry one another and call on one another's strengths. The grief support group becomes a means of sharing both weaknesses and strengths, sadnesses and joys, memories and hopes. This process enables the reentry into living that is the goal of the grief group.

All of us like to be in control of our lives and this is one reason death is so hard for us. We are totally out of control—we cannot stop death, nor can we stop the hurt and pain a death brings to those of us left behind. We cannot pretend the pain away. If we live and love we do not have a choice about experiencing the death of one we love; however, we do have a choice about *how* we experience that death. We can choose a living death for ourselves, refusing to go on with life, or we can grow through our grief and gain new meaning in our life. The bereaved can come to understand that the depth of the pain is a reflection of the capacity to love. With this kind of openness to the pain of loss, we may be able to come to a deeper appreciation of life and live more fully in the here and now, reaching out to those around us—touching and being touched.

Viktor Frankl writes, "Everything can be taken from a man but one thing: the last of the human freedoms—to choose one's attitude in any given set of circumstances, to choose one's own way."[1] This is certainly true of grief—we do not have a choice about whether we grieve, but we do have a choice about how we grieve. It is to enable this task of grieving that a grief support group is set up. The support group can enable its members to grow through their grieving.

A grief support group can help persons grieve in ways that are positive and life enhancing. Sorrow is painful alone but when shared with others it becomes more endurable. In the group the griever finds others who understand and are willing and able to bear some of the burden. Sharing deep hurt and pain brings a closeness that is not often found.

How to Begin a Grief Group

It is exciting to find churches becoming more interested in reaching out to persons who are bereaved. In the past when there was a death, the community in general would reach out to the grieving family. In our more mobile society, those who are grieving very often do not have roots in a community; they are not sustained by an ongoing and interconnected life. The church can provide this community when it is most needed.

When there is a death, the basic issues of our faith are raised—"Why did this happen to me?" "Why did God do this to me?" "I can't believe in a God that would allow this kind of tragedy." The church can allow these issues to be raised and worked through. Grieving people need to be able to verbalize their anger at God in order to work through this anger and become reconciled. What better place for this to take place than in a grief support group in the church community? In my work in such groups, I find that these faith issues are raised in many different ways—people need to be encouraged to express these faith questions and explore them. There are no pat answers, but each person can be helped to come up with his or her personal answers. The interaction within the group brings growth for each individual.

The first step for the church that wants to offer the kind of structured grief support group outlined in this chapter is to find co-facilitators. At least one of these persons should be trained professionally in group dynamics skills and have a solid knowledge of the grief process through personal and professional experience. The other co-facilitator can be a professional or a lay person sensitive to the issues of loss. The group outlined in this chapter combines the self-help concept with the structure provided by professional leadership. It is not a therapy group, but a support group.

The next step is to offer the group to individuals in your church and community. This can be done by letter to those you know have had a death in the family and also by placing a short article in the local newspaper. It is important to give the same information in the article and in the letter to individuals. Let people know why you are forming the group and what can happen in the group. In the letter, ask the individual to send in an application form, so you will know how many are planning to attend.

Screening for the group is important and should be done by the co-facilitators. When you advertise by newspaper and word of mouth, people whom you don't know may apply. For these persons, I would set up a personal interview. Do not screen too strictly because mixture in the group is important. However, if you find that someone is an alcoholic and receiving no help with the problem, you may want to refer the person to AA or another alcoholic treatment program. In the same manner, if someone is psychotic and needs much more than a grief support group, then this person should be referred. It may be that you will not discover these difficulties until the group is in progress. However, the support from the group may enable such persons to take steps to get outside help that they may not have taken on their own. I would suggest never telling someone they can't attend the group unless there is reason to believe they will harm someone else in the group or harm themselves by their participation—and I include emotional as well as physical harm. Some people are not emotionally capable of taking part in a group, and they should be screened out and referred to other organizations where they can receive the help they need.

Composition of the Group

A group works to the best advantage if there are five to ten members, plus two co-facilitators. I mentioned earlier that a mixture of people is acceptable. The mixture could include both sexes, different religious backgrounds, different types of survivors (widows, siblings, adult children, friends, widowers, spouses, parents, etc.), persons experiencing different kinds of death (long illness, suicide, accident, natural death), and persons who are at different points in their grief (2 months after the death, 6 months, 2 years). These differences will provide new learnings for everyone involved—different perspectives bring new understandings.

There are also advantages to having a group made up of survivors of similar kinds of deaths, or of widows and widowers; however, in a church community this might entail a long wait. I would not wait, but start a group with the mixture. On the other hand, if you find you have enough widows and widowers for one group and enough survivors of other categories for another group, you could start two groups. The main point is to provide a group for persons when they need this support.

At the Hospice of Northern Virginia, we have groups

for adolescents, groups for older widows and widowers, and groups made up of some of the mixtures described above. We have had as many as four members from the same family in the same group and it worked well. There are instances where it might be better to have family members in separate groups. This can be decided by discussion in an interview with the bereaved persons.

Goals for the Grief Support Group

One goal for this kind of group is to enable the expression of grief—the living out of the emotions and feelings of the group members. Emotions are allowed, accepted, and respected. By allowing their expression, the group enables its members to accept the reality and finality of death and to live through the emotional pain experienced as a result. The life and death of the loved person is integrated by sharing memories, both good and bad.

Another goal is to help members understand the mourning process so that their suffering can be seen in the context of this process rather than as isolated, with no reference to others' grief and pain. When grieving persons find that others share the manifestations of grief which they thought they alone had, there is a sense of incredible relief: "Others too can't read or can't remember anything they read in the last hour. Others can't concentrate and are forgetful. Others cry at the slightest provocation." The members learn from their reading and from each other that this too will pass. Group members can also share their coping skills—"How can I handle depression, sadness, panic?" New coping skills can be learned from one another.

Another very important goal is to enable the members to reach out to one another, to help someone else, to begin reinvesting in life again. The new relationships developed in the group are a big step in reaching out to the world, but in a safe environment. "Entertaining in my home by myself for the first time, after having entertained as a couple through forty years of marriage, is traumatic," but when it can be done first by having the group members over for coffee, it is less threatening. Therefore the facilitators of the grief group should encourage meeting in one anothers' homes. It is good to go out to lunch before or after the group meetings, and other outings for the total group and subgroups should be arranged. Also, members should be encouraged to telephone one another during the week—the more the better.

Topics for a Grief Group

The first session should be one of getting acquainted and laying the ground rules for subsequent sessions. I usually ask the members to begin by telling the group something about themselves—job, hobby, special activity, who they live with, movies they've especially enjoyed, a special pet, or whatever they'd like to share to let others know about them. The co-facilitators take part in this sharing.

Next, I pass out a sheet of information about the group—names and telephone numbers of all the co-facilitators, the goal of the support group, topics we will cover, and rules for the group. The goal of the

group is to enable members to move toward the integration of their grief into their life and to begin reinvesting themselves in life again. The ground rules:
1. Group members are encouraged to take part in all discussions, but no one is ever forced to do so.
2. Confidentiality is absolute—personal information shared during the sessions must not be discussed outside the group.
3. Group members are encouraged to meet socially during the week. However, dating is a no-no for the duration of the group because it causes difficulties in the group process.
4. The group meets once a week for two to two and one-half hours and regular attendance is very important and expected. If members must miss, they are requested to let the group know ahead of time or to call one of the co-facilitators or members.

Everyone reads the information sheet and we discuss it. We talk about the pattern of each session—most groups enjoy having coffee and tea available, and I like an atmosphere where people help themselves whenever they want. At succeeding sessions we will have a fifteen- or twenty-minute break; this gives people a chance to talk informally.

We make a contract at this point to accept the rules as written, with whatever additions the group has made. I initially contract with the group for ten weeks and renegotiate this later if more time is needed, but a group lasts no longer than fourteen weeks. However, I encourage groups to continue meeting on their own without co-facilitators—weekly, monthly, or on whatever basis they wish. Periodically, co-facilitators are invited back to a group party or event.

During the remainder of this first session (if there is time) and the next two or three sessions, time is allocated for each member to tell his or her story of loss in great detail. Other members may ask questions to understand each person's loss and pain. These sessions are filled with tears and hurt as everyone reexperiences his or her own loss and also experiences the others' losses. I never cut these stories short, because it is in these sharing sessions that the group members are able to externalize some of their pain and hurt. They also hurt with one another, and a sense of trust and a mutuality of respect is built—members begin to see themselves as a part of other people again, rather than as cut off and alone in their grief. They realize that others are grieving too.

I try never to end a session without a hug time—grieving persons are lonely persons and need physical hugging. As co-facilitator I am in a position to give them permission to hug, and they are then able to give to each other through hugging. We often have two or three rounds of hugs per session.

In the first session I ask if anyone minds giving his or her address and phone number to everyone else in the group. I have never yet had anyone who wanted the address and phone number withheld. At the second session, I hand each member a typed list of addresses and phone numbers. This encourages members to begin contacting one another during the week. New members are permitted to join the group during the first two sessions but after that the group is closed and no new members are accepted.

The first or second week I give a homework assignment: Each person is to write down his or her individual goals during the group sessions. I ask the members to think of their goals as "What I want to accomplish in this group" or "Things I'd like to change during this group." I ask them to make the goals as concrete as they can—often they are desires such as: "I want to make one new friend in this group," or "I want to be able to invite someone over for dinner," or "I want to learn to go out to eat by myself," or "I want to hurt less." We go over the goals in the next group session and then I collect them to use in the last session as part of each member's personal evaluation. In the final session each person reads his or her goals to the group and we discuss whether or not the person has accomplished those goals or has only begun to accomplish them and needs to continue. Sometimes the goals are no longer significant; there are other things that have emerged as much more important. This gives each member a chance to evaluate his or her own progress in the group and in grieving generally, and also to receive other members' perceptions of that progress.

The next session or two are devoted to "Sharing my loved person who has died." The homework assignment for this session is to bring a picture of the dead person or some other memento that will tell the group about the person and about the relationship shared. Group members have brought bowling trophies, résumés, rings, pictures, and a variety of other things to share. These sessions are times where members learn about the role changes that have occurred in one another due to the death. They are encouraged to ask questions—to ask about the good times and the difficult times in the relationship, to discover from one another the roles that are now different: "He always did the grocery shopping and I can't bear to go to the grocery now"; "She did all the cooking and I can't seem to get up the courage to begin this by myself"; "I can't get my checkbook to balance—he always paid all the bills and kept the checkbook"; and so on. Group members can begin to see ways they can help one another through some very difficult new learnings.

The next session is one of understanding the grief process and the emotions involved. I use handouts from a variety of authors showing the grief cycle, the different tasks of grieving, and the emotions and feelings involved in each. After a co-facilitator discusses the grief process, group members are encouraged to point out where they feel they are in this cycle and to talk about their emotions and feelings. This is a tool with which each member can analyze his or her position in the process and be helped to understand the emotional ups and downs. With knowledge comes power and control. Part of the goal of the group is to give the members tools and knowledge whereby they can feel they have more control.

At the end of this session I assign homework for the next meeting. Each member is to think about and write out three things:
1. Things I feel angry about that happened during the illness and death.
2. Things I feel good about that happened during the illness and death—things I'm glad I did and said.

3. Things I wish I'd said or done differently—things I regret having done or said during the illness and death.

The next session is built around sharing these feelings. The members give forgiveness and understanding to one another during this session. Often several persons will regret similar things and will have similar angers and similar things they are proud of having said or done. These three questions can certainly be adapted to include persons grieving over different kinds of deaths—sudden death, suicide, or other death.

The next session will usually be on "How I wish to memorialize my loved one." In this session we talk about visiting the cemetery—how often we visit, and its meaning for each person. We talk about special holidays and the ways in which we may remember. Some persons have found that creating a scrapbook of mementos to pass on to grandchildren is a nice way to remember. We talk about gifts to special organizations, headstones to be put in place, ashes to be placed somewhere. One family memorialized their grandmother at Christmas—each family member bought or made a special ornament for the tree in her memory.

Throughout the group sessions I utilize poems about death, loss, life, and pain, which I have gathered from a variety of places. Often poetry can express feelings in a much more poignant way than other words. I sometimes ask the group members to write their own poetry. For most people this is a totally foreign concept. However, if given easy guidelines, they're usually willing to try. The following little

A GRIEF SUPPORT GROUP

poems came from the last group I met with. The directions were that the first line of all the poems was to be *Group,* meaning this group. They were then to have a second line made up of two words, a third line of three words, a fourth line of two words, and a fifth and final line of one word, a synonym for *group*. The poems were to tell about their group and what it meant to them. After many protests that they couldn't do this, here is the result, written by members of the Afternoon Grief Group, December 7, 1982.

Group
Open Frank.
Friendly understanding Nice
Great. helpful—
Friends

Group
is caring.
Group is sharing
of our
love.

Group
Friends together
sharing past–future
learning, growing
Together

Group
Nice, understanding
sympathetic, kind, patient,
sense of humor, supportive
Team

Group
caring, sharing
loving, consoling, ministering
helpful, meaningful
Friends

Group
Listening, understanding.
concern, warm, caring
coming together
Support.

Group
very friendly
lovely, lovely people
lost spouse
Supportive

Group
Warm, friendly
supportive, sometimes sad
understanding, kind
Family

Until now, the group has been working on the first two tasks of mourning: The first task is to accept the reality of the death; the second task is to experience and share the hurt and pain. It is at this point that we turn specifically to the third task: to adjust to an environment in which the deceased is missing.[2] In previous sessions we have touched on this topic, but in this session we concentrate on it. We talk specifically about changes each person needs to make and must make in order to adjust to the new life, as well as changes each person wants to make.

The homework given the previous session was for each person to think about his or her own personal "gonna do" list. Almost everyone has a mental list of things we are "gonna do" someday. I asked the members to remember this list and to jot things down during the week as they thought of them. I also asked them to make a running list of things they now find they must do which were previously done by the deceased person. This list inevitably leads into a discussion of such things as learning to pay bills on time, balancing checkbooks, making sure the car is in good repair, buying groceries and preparing meals, preparing income-tax forms. In talking about these things, various group members share things they have discovered that help them in these new tasks, and they also teach one another skills they already know. We talk about the frustrating part of having to learn new things, but we also talk about the flip side, the sense of independence that comes from learning new skills and realizing "I can take care of myself." There is definitely a sense of real satisfaction, even though the new learnings were forced on one by a death.

A GRIEF SUPPORT GROUP

One of the inevitable questions raised in this session is the fear that there is now "No one to take care of me if I get sick." This is especially true for the elderly widow or widower, but it is a question for anyone whose spouse has died. The reality of our own personal death comes into sharper focus with each death we experience. I feel strongly that this is an idea that needs to be explored and the group is certainly a good place to do this. Members help one another think through options and possibilities. With the elderly members of the group, we have visited senior citizen housing and gathered information that will help in future planning. Always, we talk about making no quick decisions or irreversible moves while still going through mourning, but new information for later decisions doesn't hurt. It gives many members the sense that there are places for them when they can no longer live independently.

We also touch on ways members are changing their lives now, specifically because of the death—and one of these is often the changing of furniture in the house. Many persons find that life alone, or without the deceased person, means they can have the house the way they want it now. One group member expressed this:

> I have to get Fred off my back. He's dead and gone, and I have to stop always thinking about how he'd feel about this and that. I want to begin thinking about how *I* feel and what *I* want. Fred always kept the car spotless, and I have been, but recently I realized I don't have to. I don't care if the car's dirty or not. I can even allow the house to be messy. I can leave my craft projects out around the house

because I enjoy the mess, and Fred isn't here to be upset about it. I need to think about *me*—not about *we*.

When I heard that woman say this, I felt like shouting for joy because she had really accomplished a lot of her grieving work and was on her way to her new life, separate from Fred.

We all compromise when we live and share with others, and certainly in any good marriage, both persons compromise at certain points. Part of what we can regain after a death are those things we would do or have if we were separate from our friend, child, spouse, sibling, and so on. This does not mean we would choose this if we had the choice; it only means that we can find some positive sides to our loss. I know the woman above would have chosen to continue to live with Fred (no doubt about this), but because she did not have the choice, she was beginning to seek out some of the things she could feel good about, now that she was completely cut off from Fred.

As we discuss the "gonna do" lists—the lists of things we have wanted to do but never felt we had time to accomplish—we talk about why we have not done them; whether they are things that could be tried now; or whether they should stay as "gonna dos." This has led to a variety of interesting happenings. One woman who had always wanted to take piano lessons used her husband's insurance money to purchase a piano and begin her lessons. She was at the point in her grieving when she could laugh and enjoy the fact that he would "turn over in his grave" if he knew, because he'd always been very tight with money and felt a piano and lessons were extravagances. She could also share this joke with her daughter—both mother and daughter had loved the man deeply, but were also very aware of the limits he had placed on them.

Group members have encouraged one another to take art lessons, to go on a trip to visit a friend, to go to a special restaurant, or to do whatever it is that each person would like to do. They give one another permission to enjoy life again and support one another in their reaching out to enjoy.

Near the end of this session, I like to encourage group members to begin connecting to their communities and neighborhoods again in ways they had abandoned because of the death and grieving, or even in new ways that might be helpful now. We talk about neighbors and friends they have lost contact with, church activities they used to be involved in, senior citizens centers, mental health centers, recreation programs, art programs, community college courses, and so on.

Often members talk about sleeping difficulties and/or relaxation problems. I take time to discuss the need for regular medical checkups, but also the need for regular exercise. We talk about ways to learn more about exercise and relaxation—in most communities there are many classes in these areas.

In the next to last session, we further explore what Worden calls the fourth and final task of mourning: the task of withdrawing emotional energy from the deceased and reinvesting it in other relationships. Worden seems to be saying this energy is to be reinvested in only one other relationship, but I view this issue more broadly. The group process that has already been taking place results in withdrawing emotional energy from the deceased and reaching out to invest this in new friends and fellow travelers. If up to this point the group process has worked in this area, then I believe this fourth task has begun. Group members have invested much emotional energy in one another and each has gained. This does not require that these friendships continue, although they may, but it does provide a bridge by which group members begin to reinvest themselves in living relationships.

In this session, we talk about the fears that need to be overcome before a person can take the steps to again invest in close relationships with either the same or the opposite sex. Many persons have a deeply buried sense that if they begin to feel less attached to the deceased, they are dishonoring the memory; this is sometimes the cause of continued grieving: Many of us feel that the person lives in our grieving, and if we stop grieving we will forget. Being able to discuss this together helps us realize that we won't forget. To work through and end our grief is not to forget, but to remember without the incredible existential pain. To reinvest emotions into our own life and into living others will not destroy our memories of the dead.

Another important fear explored in this session is the fear that "if I commit myself to a new relationship, it too might end—that person might die, too." This is a well-grounded fear, and the key question is whether life without risk and love is worth living. Too often when we think of reinvestment, we only think of remarriage, but there are many kinds of relationships and many kinds of love. Some group members have reinvested themselves in volunteer work where they reach out to a variety of persons and risk loving in a less romantic, but nevertheless committed sense.

It is important to explore a variety of ways to reinvest oneself—commitments to volunteer activities in hospitals, children's homes, and so on; reaching out to meet new persons through church, clubs, community groups; building better relationships with those we already know and are connected with.

One of the issues that inevitably comes up in this session is the better chance men have to remarry because of the large numbers of widows as compared to widowers. This is definitely true, but hiding behind statistics does not allow for the openness to meet and experience new friendships. I try to maintain an up-to-date list of organizations for single men and women which is given out at this session. I ask anyone who tries any of the groups on the list or finds new groups to let me know how it worked out. In this way I can add to and/or delete as time goes on. This list includes many church-sponsored singles organizations. I have also found through group members that Parents Without Partners has activities for senior-citizen singles as well as for young single parents.

The last session of the group is usually a potluck dinner in one of the members' homes. At this time, as stated earlier, I pass out the list of goals each person wrote in the second session. Each person reads his or her goals aloud and discusses how these goals have been met, have begun to be met, or have changed. Then group members give feedback and offer their perceptions of each person's progress during the weeks the group has functioned. The co-facilitators also give feedback at this time. Sometimes there is need for further discussion with one or more of the members privately, and I schedule a time for this outside the group. This is done if I feel the persons need some further intervention in their life at this time, or if there are any other concerns I feel need to be expressed.

At this final session, I also ask that each member fill out an evaluation sheet about the group.[3] I utilize the input from these evaluations for future group planning.

Then I suggest that if the group wants to continue meeting periodically that is fine, but I can no longer be involved on a regular basis. Sometimes the group will set up a meeting time a month later, other times not. Some groups have continued to meet periodically while others have not met further. This is really up to the group. However, I believe that every group we have had at the Hospice of Northern Virginia has helped to develop friendships that have continued.

During the evaluation session in a recent group, one member summarized where she was at the end of the group: "When I started this group, I had only a past; now I have a present which I live each day, and I can look forward to my future."

Notes

1. Viktor E. Frankl, *Man's Search for Meaning* (New York: Washington Square Press, 1963), p. 104.
2. William J. Wordon, *Grief Counseling and Grief Therapy: A Handbook for the Mental Health Practitioner* (New York: Springer Publishing Co., 1982). The first chapter discusses the four tasks of mourning, and I have found this helpful in seeing the tasks of the grief group process.
3. I use an evaluation form I have adapted from Alice S. Demi, *Bereavement Support Groups: Leadership Manual* (Englewood, Calif.: Grief Education Institute, 1981), pp. 59-60. I wish to extend my thanks and appreciation for this useful manual. It provides many helpful ideas.

Epilogue

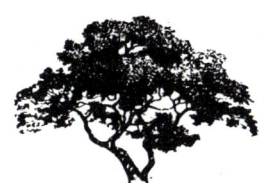

All living things eventually die. That is nature's way of keeping an ecological balance upon earth. However, the knowledge that we will die makes human beings unique. That foreknowledge also makes us anxious and fearful of the future. In recent decades much stress has been placed on the advance of medical knowledge and the health care system or the acute hospital. In this book, however, we have focused on the quiet revolution by which the hospice and lay volunteer movement is changing the care of the dying and the bereaved. People do not need a hospital in which to die; they can more comfortably die at home.

Hospice workers have made us aware of the needs of the dying: relief from pain; and a quiet place in familiar surroundings with their families, where they may spend their last days. Psychiatrists have also made us aware of the normal cycle of grief which persons go through when they lose a loved one. The need for another person to be present during that grieving has been amply demonstrated. And that person need not be a professional, but can be an especially sensitive and caring lay person.

This book has been written to help raise the consciousness of laypeople who many times have been on the fringes of caring ministry. Enabling such persons to understand the needs of the dying person and the bereaved family, as well as the church's teaching regarding the end of life and its sorrows—these represent first steps. Training laity for their legitimate ministry as care-givers in one-to-one counseling, in bereavement groups, and in death and dying seminars is a necessary second step.

Those of us involved in writing this book have confronted the death of significant persons over the period the manuscript was in process. We were reminded again that the counselor's own grief can get in the way of the helping process. William J. Wordon has listed three ways one's personal grief can block helping the grief stricken:[1]

1. If the loss experienced by the bereaved is similar to the loss in our own life.
2. If our anxiety about a possible death in our own family makes working with the bereaved difficult.
3. If we are uncomfortable with the inevitability of our own death.

The counselor needs to attend to his or her own grief before becoming a useful care-giver.

We have attempted to put the care of the dying and the bereaved within the larger context of the Christian faith. If we appear sensitive to the pain of death and the wounds of grief, that sensitivity comes from first-hand experience. Such loss should not make us bitter or afraid to face the future. Within the Christian faith we have the assurance of being within God's care no matter what we face. It is in that faith that we offer this handbook to you, knowing that your caring ministry will strengthen you against any eventuality.

Note

1. William J. Wordon, *Grief Counseling and Grief Therapy: A Handbook for the Mental Health Practitioner* (New York: Springer Publishing Co., 1982), pp. 107-8.

A Living Will

INSTRUCTIONS FOR MY CARE
IN THE
EVENT OF TERMINAL ILLNESS

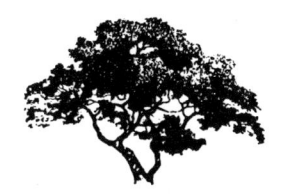

--- ... ---

My faith affirms that life is a gift of God and that physical death is a part of life, the completed stage of a person's development. My faith assures me that even in death there is hope and the sustaining grace and love of God. Because of my belief, I wish this statement to stand as the testament of my wishes.

--- ... ---

I, _____, request that I be fully informed as my death approaches. If possible, I wish to participate in decisions regarding my medical treatment and the procedures that may be used to prolong my life. If there is no reasonable expectation of my recovery from physical or mental disability, I direct my physician and all medical personnel not to prolong my life by artificial or mechanical means. I direct that I receive pain and symptom control. However, this is not a request that direct intervention be taken to shorten my life.

This decision is made after consideration and reflection. I direct that all legal means be taken to support my choice. In the carrying out of my will as stated, I release all physicians and other health personnel, all institutions and their employees, and all members of my family from legal culpability and responsibility.

Signed _____

Date _____

Witnessed By:

_____

_____

Sign and date before two witnesses. This is to insure that you signed of your own free will and not under any pressure. If you have a doctor, give him or her a copy for your medical file and discuss it to make sure she or he is in agreement. Give copies to those most

A LIVING WILL

likely to be concerned if the time comes when you can no longer take part in decisions for your own future. Discuss your intentions with them and enter their names on the original copy of the Living Will. Keep the original nearby, easily and readily available. It is a good idea to look it over once a year; redate it and initial the new date to make it clear that your wishes are unchanged.

The form of living will shown here is available from the American Protestant Hospital Association, 1701 E. Woodfield Rd., Schaumburg, IL 60195. Somewhat different forms are available from the Catholic Hospital Association, St. Louis, MO 63104, and from Concern for Dying, 250 West 57th Street, New York, NY 10019.

Bibliography

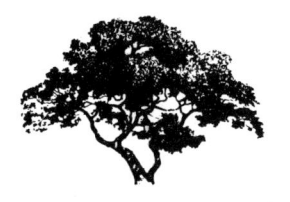

Autobiographies

Alsop, Stewart. *Stay of Execution: A Sort of Memoir.* Philadelphia: J. B. Lippincott Co., 1973.

Caine, Lynn. *Widow.* New York: William Morrow & Sons, 1974.

Cousins, Norman. *Anatomy of an Illness as Perceived by the Patient.* New York: W. W. Norton & Co., 1979.

D'Arcy, Paula. *Song for Sarah.* Wheaton, Ill.: Harold Shaw Publishers, 1979.

Evans, Jocelyn. *Living with a Man Who Is Dying: A Personal Memoir.* New York: Taplinger, 1971.

Gunther, John. *Death Be Not Proud.* New York: Harper & Row, 1949.

Lewis, C. S. *A Grief Observed.* New York: Seabury Press, 1961.

Phipps, Joyce. *Death's Single Privacy.* New York: Seabury Press, 1974.

Pincus, Lily. *Death and the Family.* New York: Random House, 1976.

Smith, Bradford. *Dear Gift of Life*. Lebanon, Penna.: Pendle Hill Publishers, 1965.

Smith, JoAnn Kelly. *Free Fall*. Valley Forge, Penna.: Judson Press, 1975.

Religious Views

Boros, Ladislaus. *The Mystery of Death*. New York: Herder & Herder, 1965.

———. *Living in Hope*. New York: Image Books, Doubleday & Co., 1973.

Bultmann, Rudolph. *Life and Death*. London: A. & C. Black, 1965.

Evely, Louis. *In the Face of Death*. New York: Seabury Press, 1979.

Lewis, C. S. *The Problem of Pain*. London: Fontana Press, 1940. New York: Macmillan Publishing Co., 1962. Paperback.

Linn, Mary Jane, and Dennis, Matthew. *Healing the Dying*. New York: Paulist Press, 1979.

Thielicke, Helmut. *Death and Life*. Philadelphia: Fortress Press, 1970.

Wolff, Pierre. *May I Hate God*. New York: Paulist Press, 1979. Paperback.

Pastoral Care

Bane, Donald, and Kutscher, Austin H., eds. *Death and Ministry*. New York: Crossroads Books, Seabury Press, 1975.

Bowers, Margaretta K., et al. *Counseling the Dying*. New York: Jay Aronson, 1975.

Fairbanks, Rollin J. "Ministering to the Dying." *Journal of Pastoral Care* 2 (1948): 6-14.

Nighswonger, Carl A. "Ministering to the Dying." *Bulletin of the American Protestant Hospital Association* 34 (November 2, 1970): 117-24.

Nouwen, Henri. *In Memorium*. Notre Dame, Ind.: Ave Maria Press, 1980.

———. *Wounded Healer*. Garden City, N.Y.: Doubleday & Co., 1972.

Reeves, Robert B., Jr., et al., eds. *Pastoral Care of the Dying and Bereaved: Selected Readings*. New York: Health Sciences Publication, 1973.

Soulen, Richard, ed. *Care for the Dying.* Atlanta: John Knox Press, 1975.

Bereavement

Jackson, Edgar N. *Understanding Grief.* Nashville: Abingdon Press, 1957.

Parkes, Colin Murray. *Bereavement: Studies of Grief in Adult Life.* New York: International University Press, 1972.

Schoenberg, Bernard, et al., eds. *Anticipatory Grief.* New York: Columbia University Press, 1974.

Hospice Care

Craven, Joan, and Wald, Florence. "Hospice Care for Dying Patients." *American Journal of Nursing* (October 1975): 1816-22.

Dobihal, Edward F., Jr. "Talk or Terminal Care." *Connecticut Medical Journal* 38/9 (July 1974): 364-67.

Dobihal, Shirley V. "Hospice: Enabling a Patient to Die at Home." *American Journal of Nursing* 80/8 (August 1980).

Hospice Volunteers: A Guide for Training. Boonton Township, N.J.: Riverside Hospice, Division of Riverside Hospital, 1980.

Lack, Sylvia A. "Hospice—A Concept of Care in the Final Stage of Life." *Connecticut Medicine* 43/6 (June 1979).

Lack, Sylvia, and Lamerton, Richard. *The Hour of Our Death.* London: Chapman Press, 1975.

Lamerton, Richard. *Care of the Dying.* London: Priory Press, 1973.

Martinson, Ida Marie. *Home Care for the Dying Child: Professional and Family Perspectives.* New York: Appleton-Century-Crofts, 1976.

Rossman, Parker. *Hospice.* New York: Association Press, 1977.

Saunders, Cicely. *Care of the Dying.* London: Macmillan & Co., 1959.

―――. "Death and Responsibility: A Medical Director's View." *Psychiatric Opinion* 3/4 (August 1966): 28-34.

―――. "The Management of Terminal Illness." *Hospital Medicine* (December 1966): 225-28; (January 1967): 317-20; (February 1967): 433-36.

―――. "A Patient." *Nursing Times* (March 31, 1961).

———. "The Treatment of Intractable Pain in Terminal Cancer." *Proceedings of the Royal Society of Medicine* 56/3 (March 1963): 191-97.

———. "Watch with Me." *Nursing Times* (November 25, 1965).

———, ed. *The Management of Terminal Disease.* Chicago: Year Book of Medical Publication, 1979.

Stoddard, Sandol. *The Hospice Movement: A Better Way of Caring for the Dying.* New York: Stein & Day, 1978.

Twycross, R. G. "Principles and Practise of the Relief of Pain in Terminal Cancer." *Update, From the Postgraduate Center.* Oxford University (July 1972).

Ethics

Beauchamp, Tom L., and Childress, James F. *Principles of Biomedical Ethics.* New York: Oxford University Press, 1979.

The Hastings Center Report. Hastings-On-Hudson, N.Y. Most issues.

Ramsey, Paul. *The Patient as Person.* New Haven: Yale University Press, 1970.

Veatch, Robert. *Death, Dying, and the Biological Revolution: Our Last Quest for Responsibility.* New Haven: Yale University Press, 1976.

Weir, Robert F., ed. *Ethical Issues in Death and Dying.* New York: Columbia University Press, 1977.

Children

Anthony, Sylvia. *The Child's Discovery of Death.* New York: Harcourt, Brace & Co., 1940.

Gordon, Audrey K., and Dennis, Klass. *They Need to Know: How to Teach Children About Death.* Englewood Cliffs, N.J.: Prentice-Hall, 1979.

Grollman, Earl A. *Talking About Death: A Dialogue Between a Parent and a Child.* Boston: Beacon Press, 1970.

Hermann, Nina. *Go Out in Joy.* Atlanta: John Knox Press, 1977.

LeShan, Eda. *Learning to Say Goodbye: When a Parent Dies.* New York: Macmillan Publishing Co., 1978.

General—Death and Dying

Becker, Ernest. *The Denial of Death.* New York: Free Press, 1973.

Brim, Orville G., Jr., et al., eds. *The Dying Patient.* New York: Russell Sage Foundation, 1970.

Glaser, Barney G., and Strauss, Anselm R. *Awareness of Dying*. Chicago: Aldine Publishing Co., 1965.

Kübler-Ross, Elisabeth. *On Death and Dying*. New York: Macmillan Co., 1969.

———. *Death: The Final Stage of Growth*. Englewood Cliffs, N.J.: Prentice-Hall, 1975.

Neale, Robert E. *The Art of Dying*. New York: Harper & Row, 1971.

Pincus, Lily. *Death and the Family*. New York: Random House, 1976.

Film Resources

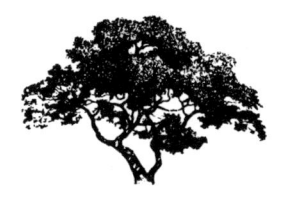

Hospice—An alternative way to care for the dying. Produced by the National Hospice Organization to create community awareness and knowledge of the hospice concept.

    Billy Budd Films, Inc.   Sale $350.00
    235 E. 57th Street
    New York, NY 10022   Rental $ 35.00

As Long as There Is Life—Nothing in this film was staged. It is a *cinema verite* of the Forest family. Pat Forest felt that if the story of her illness and death could benefit others, then this was what she wished as her legacy. Dick, her husband, and Rick and Mark, her young sons, agreed. Their moving story shows how the Connecticut Hospice Home Care Team shared in their life. An excellent discussion guide accompanies this film, and a transcription of the dialogue is available on request. C-40 min.

    John Abbott   Sale $405.00
    The Connecticut Hospice, Inc. (includes $10 shipping)

61 Burban Drive   Rental $ 55.00
Branford, CT 06405   (includes $10 shipping)

How Could I Not Be Among You?—A film about Ted Rosenthal, a poet who comes to grips with acute leukemia and the fact of his death. It explores the ways he coped with his feelings and gained a new kind of freedom.   C-28 min.

Benchmark Films, Inc.   Sale $410.00
145 Scarborough Road
Briarcliff Manor, NY 10510   Rental $ 40.00

Whose Life Is It Anyway?—A film of a young paraplegic's decision to forego recommended treatment and die. Illustrates the personal and professional struggles in making decisions and determining responsibility.   C-53 min.

Eccentric Circle Cinema Workshop   Sale $650.00
Box 4085
Greenwich, CT 06830   Rental $ 60.00

Essie—A documentary by Gerald Wenner. Portrays a young woman with cancer and her struggle to take responsibility for her illness, her life, her death.   C-55 min.

Filmakers Library, Inc.   Sale $750.00
133 E. 58 St.
New York, N.Y. 10022   Rental $ 75.00

The Death of a Newborn Child—An interview with parents of newborns. Shows the tragedy of grief.   C-33 min.

New England Institute   Sale $350.00
Beacon Ave.
Boston, Mass.   Rental $ 40.00

Do I Really Want to Die?—Discussion among persons who thought about and attempted suicide. They speak in a frank, penetrating way of their behavior and the feelings that led up to the suicide attempt.

Polymorph Films, Inc.   Sale $135.00
118 South St.
Boston, MA 02111   Rental $ 40.00

Soon There Will Be No More of Me—Documents a young wife and mother stricken with cancer and her determination to write a book that will communicate her experience to the world and to her young daughter, who will someday want to know the mother she cannot remember.   C-10 min.

Churchill Films   Sale $130.00
662 North Robertson Blvd.
Los Angeles, CA 90069   Rental $ 15.00

To Die Today—Presents Elisabeth Kübler-Ross' theories and their humanizing effect on care of the terminally ill.   B/W-50 min.

Filmakers Library, Inc.   Sale $500.00
133 E. 58 St.
New York, NY 10022   Rental $ 50.00

We're Not Alone—Reactions of three women to loss of their spouses.

Learning Resource Center
UConn Health Center
Farmington, CT 06032   Rental only $ 10.00

Widows—Frank comments by recently widowed women. Describes the stresses of widowhood and single parenthood and suggests strategies for intervention.   B/W-41 min.

U. of California Extension Media Center
Berkeley, CA 94720   Rental $ 19.00

When a Child Dies—A moving film of three families that lost young children and the effect it had on the parents, siblings, and their life together. The film involves the viewers and stimulates discussion of a difficult topic. The National Funeral Directors Association helped produce this film; a local funeral director must help you secure it for single viewing.

National Funeral Directors Association
135 W. Wells Street
Milwaukee, WI 53203   Sale $225.00

Until I Die—Elisabeth Kübler-Ross explains her work with the terminally ill and examines the five stages through which the patients progress after learning of their impending deaths. A patient interview and a follow-up conference with staff members are also shown.   C-30 min.

American Journal of Nursing
% Association Films, Inc.
866 Third Ave.
New York, NY 10022

You See, I've Had a Life—When the teenager in this film is diagnosed as having leukemia, his family choose not to hide it, but attempt to share and face the experience with him.   B/W-30 min.

Eccentric Circle Cinema Workshop   Sale $290.00
Box 4085
Greenwich, CT 06830   Rental $ 29.00

Media Guide on Death and Dying, published by Biomedical Communications, 750 Third Ave., New York, NY 10017, lists some of these and also many other films.

Index

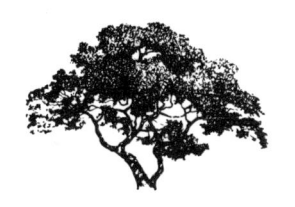

Acceptance
  by bereaved, 100-101, 112, 194; of life journey, 91-92, 94; by terminally ill, 66, 69-70, 103
Anger
  at God, 66-68; in grief work, 47-48
Anticipatory grief, 104-5
Anxiety, 15, 22-24, 40-41, 47-48, 81, 117, 164-66

Bargaining by terminally ill, 66-68

Becker, Ernest, 16
Bereaved, the
  fears in, 195; goal-setting for, 194-99; isolation of, 180-81; motivation of, 143-45, 151-53; needs of, 39-53, 130-31, 149-50; pain of, 174-75
Bereavement. *See* Grief; Grief work
Between Man and Man (Buber), 89-90
Blockage of grief care, 202-3
Body, awareness of, 19-20, 34

Bowen, Murray, 50-52
Bowlby, John, 40-41
Buber, Martin, 89-90
Butler, Robert, 92

Care-giver, accreditation of, 156
Care-giver, primary, 131-34
Care-givers, lay
  continuing education for, 158-59; motivation of, 63; priestly function of, 93-94; screening of, 132-33; for terminally ill and bereaved, 10-11, 122-23; training of, 130-59
Care-givers, pastoral, 94-95, 114-28
  goals of, 60-61, 73; in minority churches, 74-75; motivation of, 63; qualifications for, 63-64; training of, 63-75; visits by, 72-75. *See also* Care-givers, lay; Pastoral care
Care-givers, professional
  control by, 63; role in home care, 27-28. *See also* Nurses; Physicians
Caring
  in animals, 87; in ministry, 117, 120, 164-69; as scriptural themes, 89-91; societal structures for, 87-88
Christ. *See* Jesus
Christian faith, message of, 77-95, 117
Church
  and response to need, 114-28; and role in care of dying and grieving, 10-11, 54-76; and teaching about death, 77-95. *See also* Church, local
Church, local
  and care for bereaved, 181; caring ministry in, 117, 164-69; consciousness raising in, 167-69; and death-related issues, 163-67
Clemons, Barbara, 93-94
Cocoanut Grove fire, 44
Communication
  in family, 111-12; with family of terminally ill, 65; with terminally ill, 64-70
Compassion, 90-91
Confession of sins, 93-94
Conflict
  with community, 116-17; with physicians, 116, 121
Confrontation, training for, 139-41. *See also* Death
Congregation. *See* Church, local
Consciousness raising, 167-69
Control
  of health care, 57-60, 63; of life, 20, 26, 28-29, 60-63, 64, 182
Courage to Be (Tillich), 86-87
Creative living by terminally ill, 106-9

Death
  confrontation of, 54-55, 75, 169-72; definition of, 21; desire for, 18-19; and faith issues, 183; as normal event, 114-15; preparation for, 118; as topic for discussion, 55-56, 164-67; of the young, 174-75

INDEX

Death and Dying Seminar, 160-79
Death and the Family (Pincus), 105
Death, sudden, 13-16
Decathexis, 40, 47
Denial, 22-23, 66-67, 103-5, 141
Dependence, as condition of living, 23
Depression, 45-47, 68-69
Disorganization in grief, 42-45, 48
Dying
  acknowledgment of, 59; options for, 175-77; physical aspects of, 18-19; process of, 13, 16
Dying, the. *See* Terminally ill, the

Empathy, 89-90, 137
Erikson, Erik, 93-94
Escape of bereaved, 109-10
E.T., 85

Family
  alienation in, 86; as bereaved, 111-13; of the terminally ill, 27-28, 31, 62-65, 70-75, 97
Family balance, 41-42, 50-51, 110-11
Fear
  in bereaved, 195; of emotional reinvestment, 198-99; of pain, 24-26; of sudden death, 13-14; in terminally ill, 24-26; of terminally ill, 117
Final Payments (Gordon), 139-40

Finitude, 15-16, 49
Fowler, James, 93
Frankl, Viktor, 144-45, 182
Freud, Sigmund, 40, 42, 47
From Death Camp to Existentialism (Frankl), 144-45
Funeral, 55-56, 104, 105

God
  absence of, 79-80; anger at, 66-68; as caring, 88-89; dependence on, 32-34, 36, 37, 38; experience of, 89-90; faith in, 49; justice of, 79; presence of, 75-76; providence of, 94
Gordon, Mary, 139-40
Gospel. *See* Jesus; New Testament themes
Grief
  ambivalence of, 47-48; in childhood, 40-41, 50-52, 113; defenses against, 141; definition of, 41; depression during, 47-48; growth in, 182; nature of, 40-44, 153-56; process of, 39-40, 42-45; social needs during, 41, 46-48; stages of, 32-33, 41-52; support groups for, 180-200. *See also* Grief work
Grief, severe, referral for, 153-55
Grief work
  acceptance of death in, 100-101, 194; goal-setting in, 142-45; need for, 112-13; reorganization as a goal in, 48-52, 196-97; roles in, 137-39
Grieving. *See* Bereaved, the;

Grief; Grief work
Grieving Family, A (case study), 96-113
Growth in grief, 182
Guilt
  in family, 112; in grief, 43, 47-48, 49; at illness, 26-27, 33; for past, 92-94

Hallucinations, 46
Harvard Project, 41
Healing ministry, 122
Health care
  holistic, 11; by lay care-givers, 10-11, 122-23; orientation of, 17-19, 57; for terminally ill, 17-19, 124. *See also* Hospice movement; Hospitals
Home care
  example of, 34-36; for terminally ill, 27-32, 62-65
Hope
  modes of, 82-84, 87; as scriptural theme, 80-82, 94-95
Hospice, Inc., 116-17
Hospice movement, 10-11, 27
  church's role in, 120-22, 125, 127-28; conflict in, 116-117; definition of, 124; federal help for, 120-21; philosophy of, 161-63; planning for, 122-23, 125-28
Hospice of Northern Virginia, 184-85, 200
Hospitals
  acute, 15; church establishment of, 122; patient's loss of control in, 23-25; for terminally ill, 27-29

Illness, chronic, 17
Isolation, 86, 114-15

Jesus
  as caring, 88-90; and conquest of death, 83-84; as example, 94-95; and resurrection, 88; and stories of loss, 78-79
Job, 79, 80
John of the Cross, 80
Jung, Carl, 93

Klein, Melanie, 40
Krabill, Willard S., 114-15
Kübler-Ross, Elisabeth, 9, 13, 21, 66-67
Kushner, Harold S., 81

Last Letter to the Pebble People (Hine), 148-49
Lay care-givers. *See* Care-givers, lay
Leavetaking, 27, 30-32, 34-38
Lewis, Myrna, 92
Life Line, in Training Module, 142-43, 144
Life review, 78, 91-98, 145-46 (exercise)
Lifton, Robert J., 82-84
Lindemann, Erich, 42, 44, 45-46
Listening, 56-58, 59-60, 102, 123, 125
  training for, 138-39
Living will. *See* Will, living
Loss
  coping with, 134-37; as scriptural theme, 78-80; varieties of, 134, 172-74
Love, as basis for care, 84-90

Magno, Josefina, 10

INDEX

Maturity, 93
May, Rollo, 89
Medical advances, 15
Medicare, 121
Minister. *See* Pastor
Motivation
  of bereaved, 143-45; of lay care-givers, 63, 151-53
Mourning and Melancholia (Freud), 40

National Hospice Organization, 10
Near-death experiences, 118
New Testament themes, 88-89. *See also* Gospel; Jesus
Nuclear social unit (nonfamily), 70-71
Nurses
  in hospice movement, 126-27; as ministers, 35-36, 56. *See also* Care-givers, professional
Nursing homes, 122

Old Testament themes, 88-89

Pain
  fear of, 103; relief of, 19, 33; responsibility for, 19
Parents Without Partners, 199
Parkes, Colin Murray, 41, 44-45, 97, 109
Participation
  of family in care, 27-32, 62-65; of patient in care, 20-21, 64
Pastor, role of, 77, 166. *See also* Caregivers, pastoral; Pastoral care
Pastoral care
  of dying and grieving, 60-62; in early church, 95
Pastoral care-givers. *See* Care-givers, pastoral
Paul (apostle), 81-82
Physicians
  conflict with, 116; criteria for, 21-22; responsibility of, 58-59; role in hospice, 126-27. *See also* Care-givers, professional
Pincus, Lily, 105
Prayer
  in anxiety, 81; for healing, 101; with terminally ill, 36
Professional care-givers. *See* Care-givers, professional
Priestly function, 93-94
Progoff, Ira, 91-92
Pruyser, Paul, 81

Quinlan, Karen Ann, 58

Recathexis, 40
Reconciliation to dying, 37-38
Referral in severe grief, 153-55
Reinvestment, emotional, 197-99
Reorganization as a goal in grief, 48-52, 196-97
Resurrection, 88
Retribution, 79
Ritual Exercise, 148-49
Rituals of life, 117-18
Rogers, Carl, 150-51
Role-play for care-givers, 137-38, 139, 141, 155-56

St. Christopher's Hospice, 9, 127-28, 129
Saunders, Cicely, 9, 120, 128
Schachtel, Ernest, 81

Scriptural themes of dying and grieving, 77-95
Self-affirmation, 86-87, 90-91
Self-evaluation in grief, 146-48
Seminar on Death and Dying, 160-79
Separation and Loss (Bowlby), 40-41
Shock, 42, 43-45, 104
Smith, Bradford, 30, 54-55, 75
Social systems theory, 41-42
Social workers, 73
Stewart, Charles, 113
Sudden death, 13-16
Suffering, as scriptural theme, 79
Support groups. *See* Grief, support groups

Tabor, Eithne, 135
Teresa, Mother, 9, 91
Terminal care. *See* Care-givers, lay; Home care; Hospice movement; Hospitals; Terminally ill, the
Terminally ill, the
  emotional needs, 24-25; fears, 24-26; immediate goals, 32; isolation, 24; physical aspects, 18-19; psychological needs, 23-24; rights, 17-18, 19-22; social needs, 25-32; spiritual needs, 32-38
Thomas, Dylan, 25
Thurman, Howard, 131
Tillich, Paul, 49, 86-87
Training Module, A (for lay care-givers), 130-59

Volunteers, 11, 126-28, 133

Will, living, 59-60, 61
  example of, 205-7
Withdrawal by bereaved, 119
Wordon, William J., 197, 202-3